Bodies in Blue

UnCivil Wars

SERIES EDITORS

Stephen Berry,
University of Georgia

Amy Murrell Taylor,
University of Kentucky

ADVISORY BOARD

Edward L. Ayers,
University of Richmond
Catherine Clinton,
University of Texas at San Antonio
J. Matthew Gallman,
University of Florida
Elizabeth Leonard,
Colby College

James Marten,
Marquette University
Scott Nelson,
College of William & Mary
Daniel E. Sutherland,
University of Arkansas
Elizabeth Varon,
University of Virginia

Bodies in Blue
Disability in the Civil War North

SARAH HANDLEY-COUSINS

The University of Georgia Press   *Athens*

© 2019 by the University of Georgia Press
Athens, Georgia 30602
www.ugapress.org
All rights reserved
Set in 10.5/13 Adobe Caslon Pro by
Graphic Composition, Inc., Bogart, Georgia

Most University of Georgia Press titles are
available from popular e-book vendors.

Printed digitally

Library of Congress Cataloging-in-Publication Data

Names: Handley-Cousins, Sarah, 1984– author.
Title: Bodies in blue : disability in the Civil War north / Sarah Handley-Cousins.
Other titles: Physical wreck of his former self
Description: Athens : The University of Georgia Press, [2019] | Series: Uncivil wars |
    Revision of author's thesis (doctoral)—State University of New York at Buffalo, 2016, titled
    "A physical wreck of his former self" : gender and disability in the post Civil War north. |
    Includes bibliographical references and index.
Identifiers: LCCN 2018049579| ISBN 9780820355184 (hardcover ; alk. paper) |
    ISBN 9780820355191 (ebook)
Subjects: LCSH: Disabled veterans—United States—History—19th century. |
    United States—History—Civil War, 1861–1865—Veterans. | Masculinity—
    Social aspects—United States—19th century.
Classification: LCC E621 .H324 2019 | DDC 305.9/08097309034—dc23
LC record available at https://lccn.loc.gov/2018049579

For my mom, Debra

O you regiments so piteous, with your mortal diarrhea! with your fever!
O my land's maimed darlings! with the plenteous bloody bandage and the crutch!

—WALT WHITMAN, "A Carol of Harvest for 1867"

CONTENTS

ACKNOWLEDGMENTS   *xi*

INTRODUCTION
Disability and the American Civil War   *1*

CHAPTER 1
Gather the Invalids   *11*

CHAPTER 2
Army of the Walking Sick   *33*

CHAPTER 3
The United States Government Is Entitled to All of You   *51*

CHAPTER 4
The Disabled Lion of Union   *71*

CHAPTER 5
Man or Mercenary   *95*

CHAPTER 6
The Long, Long Years of Misery   *115*

EPILOGUE   *133*

NOTES   *137*

BIBLIOGRAPHY   *165*

INDEX   *181*

ACKNOWLEDGMENTS

This book simply would not exist without the generous intellectual, financial, and emotional support of a great many wonderful humans. I'll try to pay homage to them all, but perhaps one deserves top billing. Carole Emberton and I arrived at the University at Buffalo the same semester. She has seen me through two degrees, alternately encouraging me and holding my feet to the fire. When I told her I wanted to write about Joshua Lawrence Chamberlain, instead of laughing, Carole told me to go for it. Since then, her guidance has helped me to navigate all aspects of the writer-scholar's life. I could not have asked for a better mentor.

I am indebted to the Department of History at the University at Buffalo for a number of reasons. As a doctoral student, I received generous research funding that made all those trips to Washington, DC, and Maine possible, and travel grants allowed me to workshop ideas with a broader academic community. My colleagues have helped me to grow as a teacher and scholar. Michael Rembis and Susan Cahn patiently read draft after draft. Erik Seeman offered important insights that helped to shape chapters 2 and 3. Victoria Wolcott and Gail Radford have both been steadfast advocates, and so many others have been there with advice and warmth. I am also thankful to Susan Buttaccio, Gloria Piotrowski, and Michelle Burger for their friendship. I'm grateful to have spent so many years of my life in this intellectual community.

At my first Society of Civil War Historians meeting, I was convinced that my paper would be roundly jeered. Instead, I found a wide variety of scholars ready to answer endless questions, share research tips, give reading suggestions, dole out career advice, and offer moral support. Diane Miller Sommerville's recommendations helped me to bring the project from dissertation to manuscript, and her eagle eye improved my writing enormously. Kathryn Shively's advice helped me to think through Chamberlain's story with greater depth. Dillon Carroll and David Thomson offered much-needed encouragement that has helped me stay with this project over the years. (As a Bowdoin grad, David even gave me the inside scoop about

Chamberlain's special chair!) Others have offered their help over the years. Kelly Mezurek very generously chatted with me about the Invalid Corps and offered an advance copy of some of her work on the topic, which was indispensable. Michael Rhode kindly helped me understand Circular No. 2 and the creation of the Army Medical Museum.

I also met Matthew Hulbert at that first meeting, and he became a comrade almost immediately. I am especially indebted to Matt for putting me in touch with his editors at UnCivil Wars and the University of Georgia Press. Stephen Berry and Amy Murrell Taylor believed in this project from the very beginning—indeed, Steve took this project under his wing just weeks after I defended the dissertation, and over the years he has helped me to reconceptualize and reconfigure it into a much better work. Mick Gusinde-Duffy always had confidence in the manuscript when I was feeling defeated. I am grateful to all three, as well as to the rest of the dedicated team at the University of Georgia Press.

Many archivists and librarians kindly helped in my research. Jim Folts at the New York State Archives ushered me through the complicated process of accessing restricted asylum patient records, and he read drafts to ensure they adhered to the requirements of the New York State mental hygiene laws. Mildred Jones, volunteer archivist of the First Parish Church in Brunswick, Maine, carved time out of her day for me to peruse Rev. George Adams's diaries and gave me a tour of the beautiful church. Former Pejepscot Historical Society director Jennifer Blanchard and her staff were incredibly helpful. They even snuck me into an elementary school tour of Joshua Lawrence Chamberlain's home, which was otherwise closed for the season. The patient archivists at the National Archives in Washington, DC, and the National Museum of Health and Medicine in Silver Spring, Maryland, helped me navigate many a complicated finding aid.

When I first pitched an essay to a start-up history blog called *Nursing Clio* in 2013, little did I know that I would find some of my dearest friends: Jacqueline Antonovich, Lauren McIvor Thompson, Laura Ansley, Amelia Grabowski, Lizzie Reis, R. E. Fulton, Cassia Roth, Carrie Adkins, Averill Earls, and Adam Turner. This incredible team has taught me so much, but more importantly, its members have been a critical emotional support. I am immensely proud of the work we do and ever thankful for my colleagues' friendship.

In Buffalo, many miles from my blood family, I was blessed with friends who have become another family. All the members of our little writing group, Elisabeth George, Colin Eager, Maggie Magdalena, Kathryn Lawton, and Jake Newsome, offered extensive thoughts and revisions, read innumerable drafts, and told me which of my darlings I needed to kill. I owe many chapter titles, anecdotes, modes of analysis, and turns of phrase to them. Billy Pritchard was my very first friend in graduate school, and he acted as an ally for the better part of ten years. My co-producers on *Dig: A History Podcast* are a daily source of love and encouragement. I am deeply grateful for Marissa Rhodes's and Elizabeth Garner Masarik's friendship. I am endlessly inspired by their work ethic, creativity, and strength. Averill Earls has been a cheerleader, schemer, shoulder to cry on, candy bringer, and endless source of strength, amusement, and cheese. I'm not sure I could have done any of this without her. Homies help homies. Always.

I would be remiss if I did not thank a bevy of nannies and teachers who cared for my children while I locked myself in the office, particularly Jessica Lang, Megan Brown, and Larissa Smith, who literally made this work possible.

I have often reflected that in some way, I have been on the path to becoming a historian since I was very small. My family members, I think, knew this before I did, and each of them had a unique way of helping me to navigate that path. When I was too little to have done anything interesting at all, my grandmother declared that I would be a writer—and she was right. My grandfather gathered talismans, now lining my bookshelves, when he traveled: a shard of a tree near the Crater, a rail spike from City Point. My father gave me his copy of John Jakes's *North and South* when I was eleven and his copy of *The Killer Angels* when I was fifteen, and on nearly every vacation we dragged the rest of the family to every battlefield within driving distance. His love of the Civil War became my love of the Civil War. None of these relatives will get to read this book, but I don't believe they need to. They've been there every step of the way.

James Cousins is a life partner in the truest sense: he is my best friend, my co-parent, the love of my life. He has never doubted me for a moment, and in many ways, he has shaped his life to make my perhaps foolhardy dreams possible. For that, I am profoundly grateful. My mother has been there for every success and every heartache, with a bottle of wine and spiritual sustenance. She sees in me what I do not see in myself. This book is for her.

Finally, to Ainsley, Emma, and Zoey: never let them tell you it can't be done. It can.

Bodies in Blue

INTRODUCTION

Disability and the American Civil War

In *The March*, E. L. Doctorow's novel about William Tecumseh Sherman's Savannah campaign, army surgeon Wrede Sartorius, eager to learn in the "practicum" of carnage, takes custody of horrifically wounded corporal Albion Simms. An accidental powder explosion has driven an iron spike into Simms's skull and pierced his brain. The spike doesn't kill the corporal, but it leaves him with no memory—his consciousness resets every few seconds. Even by midsentence, Simms has forgotten the meaning of his words. The case fascinates the coldly inquisitive Sartorius, who knows the young man will certainly die, but slowly.

Rather than hospitalize him away from the front lines, the doctor brings Simms on the march so he can document his gradual but inevitable decline. Dr. Sartorius at one point describes the wound in agonizing detail to Simms, who has been strapped to a table. The young man's eyes roll in terror, and he cannot comprehend what is happening to him: "Wrede Sartorius looked into his eyes and smiled, and laid a hand on his chest. Corporal Albion Simms, he said, you will not have surgery. Your survival is something of a miracle. And that miracle is precisely what invites our examination."[1] These words—"your survival is something of a miracle" that "invites our examination"—might as easily have been said to any number of the men who survived the Civil War. Lead balls ripped through flesh and splintered bones. Cannonballs carried limbs clean away. Dysentery and typhoid and smallpox and malaria shrunk men to shadows. Survival was often a kind of miracle.

From the moment the first shattered men emerged from the smoke of the battlefield, we, like Dr. Sartorius, have been utterly transfixed. No film or television show on the war is complete without a graphic amputation, no battlefield tour quite finished without a description of the blood slick on the field hospital floor. Museum exhibitions draw patrons to gaze at partly nude soldiers displaying suppurating wounds or prosthetic limbs for the camera. There's something about the way the Civil War destroyed men's bodies that continues to draw us in.

In spite of this fascination, we still know relatively little about wartime disability—that is, while we often catch glimpses of injury and illness, few works focus specifically on the ways that impairment challenged and changed Civil War veterans. In recent years, historians have begun to look more closely at health and the body during the war, reevaluating the conflict's medical history and adding an important new dimension to our knowledge of the lives of wounded and disabled soldiers.[2] Almost all of the scholarship on Civil War disability focuses on amputation, and with good reason. Amputation was the most dramatic and obvious wound of the era, and the absence of an arm or a leg quickly symbolized the losses of the war writ large.

As powerful a cultural touchstone as a missing limb was, amputations made up only a small fraction of Civil War wounds. Almost all of the men who were discharged disabled from the Union army either suffered a trauma that did not result in amputation or succumbed to disease. While amputation certainly did raise concerns about manhood and disability, it also carried great cultural cachet. During the war, amputation became the most powerful symbol of the conflict's destructive power. Songs, poems, stories, and popular imagery all invoked missing limbs to represent the collective loss and sacrifice of Federal soldiers and the Union as a whole. Few would question a Union amputee's sacrifice and worth. Things became decidedly more muddled, however, when a soldier bore wounds that were complicated, hidden, or difficult to define. What happened when a serviceman claimed to be disabled but bore no obvious scars? How exactly might the public honor chronic diarrhea in sentimental etchings?

My aim in this book is to push us beyond Dr. Sartorius's medical fascination and toward a broader social and cultural understanding of war-related disabilities in the Civil War North. Though one or two amputees do make an appearance, this history of disability does not focus on amputation. This is not to say that amputation did not generate social anxieties or pose serious bodily challenges. Rather, as the impairment most closely associated with the war, amputation did not raise the same questions about legitimacy and worthiness as less straightforward ailments. We will instead explore the ways in which soldiers, civilians, and institutions grappled with disorders that did not easily fit into existing cultural narratives of manhood and sacrifice. Centering our attention on such bodies reveals a very different story about Civil War wounds, one where disabled soldiers were just as likely to be used, rejected, separated, and distrusted as they were to be honored.

While war wounds have often been interpreted as fitting outside of the larger narrative of disability in the United States, disability has long been relegated to the margins of Civil War history. War injuries were imbued with ideas about patriotic sacrifice. Thus, historians have concluded convincingly that some Civil War soldiers and veterans accepted their bodily losses and took pride in their pain's part in the larger conflict.[3] In addition, disabled Union veterans received financial support from the federal government in the form of pensions, a benefit many other disabled people went without.[4]

Despite attempts to transform war wounds into badges of honor, the stigma of disability and dependence remained. As we will see, concern about disability's effect on Union soldiers emerged early in the war despite rhetoric of patriotic sacrifice. The War Department immediately initiated efforts to prevent soldiers from becoming dependent paupers. After the war, while the pension system ostensibly existed to support all those disabled in the line of service, the process to obtain a pension relied on a veteran's ability to fit within the state's strict definitions of disability. As a result, many veterans struggled to convince pension bureaucrats they were, in fact, physically and morally deserving of federal support. As historian Rabia Belt succinctly notes, "Dependence trumps deservedness even with veterans."[5] The idea of patriotic sacrifice could also work against veterans, as further costs—continued military service, settling for low pension payments, even relinquishing body parts to the pursuit of medical science—were couched within the language of the duty of citizen-soldiers.

Anxieties that disabled soldiers would descend into immoral pauperism arose out of mid-nineteenth-century ideas about manhood. American masculinity in this era was multifaceted, and conceptions of manhood varied across ethnic, class, and regional lines. However, the ability to command one's body and use it in labor to maintain independence was a value shared across boundaries. Military service added further gendered expectations, such as the requirement to submit to authority and face adversity with cheerful determination. As Lorien Foote demonstrates, the Union army combined and augmented the two general categories of antebellum manhood first described by Amy Greenberg. This martial masculinity combined elements of restrained manhood, which valued temperance and self-control, with martial manhood, which emphasized dominance, strength, and violence, to create an ideological construct I refer to as the "true soldier of

Union."⁶ Ideal Union citizen-soldiers respected authority without being overly submissive. They also possessed a strong sense of duty and demonstrated bravery, stoicism, and an ability and willingness to use violence. Not all soldiers met this model, of course, but all were measured against it.

Men were also judged according to their ability to work and provide for their dependents. During the first decades of the nineteenth century, the Revolutionary principles of independence and self-sufficiency became particularly important as the growth of wage labor subordinated a significant portion of the male population to other men in the market economy. As wage earning dominated the American marketplace, dependency became more about economic independence than complete self-sufficiency. Those who could not achieve financial autonomy—nonwhites, women, children, and the disabled—became dependents. While it was natural for some (women, children, and nonwhites) to be dependent on white men, the term took on a tone of moral judgment when referring to adult males who did not fulfill their obligation to be independent or to provide.⁷ Disabled people have found myriad ways to be productive throughout history. Even so, the assumption that disability spelled a life of dependency helped to stoke fear that Union soldiers risked becoming paupers.

Maintaining self-mastery proved especially important when soldiers became veterans. As historians including Gerald Linderman and Reid Mitchell show, many Americans considered the Civil War a crucible for manhood, refining men and molding them into model citizens. Ideally, then, Union veterans were paragons of their gender. However, many of these ideal men bore impairments that made it difficult for them to adhere to masculine tenets of self-mastery and productivity, thus placing them in real danger of becoming paupers. The safety net created to prevent soldiers' and veterans' indigence, the federal pension system, also required that men demonstrate their inability to work. Soldiers had to testify that they could not meet the ideals of manhood in order to receive payments. Disabled veterans had to balance their masculinity not only with their impairment, but also with their need for pension support. Some managed these feats more successfully than others. Certain veterans failed to find a balance, struggling to find work and keep a happy home. At times, as James Marten and Jonathan Jones demonstrate, they sank into alcohol and opium addictions.⁸ Others, like James Tanner and Joshua Lawrence Chamberlain, who enjoyed political careers and fame in veteran circles, managed the balancing act with more success.

Just as veterans had vastly different experiences after the war, wounded or sick soldiers and veterans drew different conclusions from their disabilities.

Certainly, many soldiers took pride in the role their bodies had played in the Union victory. Yet as Kim Nielsen notes, pride did not save them from the dishonor, difficulty, and indignity that often accompanied disabled lives in an able-bodied world. This book is deeply influenced by the work of historians and scholars of disability. I interpret the combat wounds and sicknesses of the Civil War era through the social model, which teaches that disabilities are social and cultural constructs rather than isolated medical events. This approach opposes the medical model, which interprets disability as a condition that can and should be cured. When analyzed through the lens of the social model, a Civil War–related disability had effects far beyond the medical reality of a wound and the impairment it created.[9] Disability rendered soldiers and veterans vulnerable to the military justice system and medical authorities. It sparked distrust and disdain from the Pension Bureau and the public. Moreover, it shook families and altered imagined futures.

Approaching Civil War disability through this framework also means rejecting the narratives of overcoming and inspiration that often appear in writing about disabled people.[10] As we will see with the case of Joshua Lawrence Chamberlain, we often do not consider successful veterans disabled. Instead, we reserve the label only for those more obviously impaired or in need of greater accommodation. As a result, it can appear as if accomplishment somehow allowed disabled men to overcome or leave behind their impairments, which is, of course, impossible. At the same time, soldiers and veterans who endured extreme suffering and lived to tell about it have been held up as inspirations, men whose almost superhuman abilities allowed them to transcend impairment—Chamberlain as Civil War "supercrip." In reality, these disabled soldiers and veterans had little choice but to learn how to effectively exist within an ableist society. In some cases, they crafted personas that deflected attention from an impairment.

While these soldiers' ability to pass shielded them from the stigma of disability, it could also work against them. Court-martial boards rejected soldiers' claims of impairment, or the Pension Bureau interpreted adaptation as a sign of able-bodiedness and cut federal support. These narratives undergird a falsely dichotomous definition of disability, one in which men whose profound impairments required constant care are the only ones understood to be disabled. In contrast, men with different kinds of abilities and differences and who lived more independently are viewed as somehow nondisabled. Disability does not equal ruin and despair. Operating from that assumption flattens the richly nuanced, complicated history of Civil War disability into a dark story about bitter, broken men.[11]

Sources constitute an inherent problem in exploring the experiences of disabled soldiers. This work draws on a variety of source materials, but it relies particularly on the words of combatants and veterans themselves as recorded in pension documents, patient case files, courts-martial, and other papers. The problem is not that materials are scarce, but that they are often open to interpretation. Able-bodied individuals in positions of authority have long possessed the power to define disability. Officers, surgeons, and pension bureaucrats scrutinized soldiers' and veterans' bodies, questioning—and often rejecting—their own accounts of pain or sickness. One can feel reasonably sure that a pension document asserting that a veteran lost a leg is truthful, but the testimony of men whose ailments were difficult to characterize or diagnose may raise questions. In documents in which a soldier described a bout of diarrhea from decades earlier or tried to get out of court-martial charges by claiming ill health, it is tempting to look for reasons he might have exaggerated or feigned symptoms, especially when doctors and officers challenged soldiers' claims. In this book, I choose to take soldiers and veterans at their word about their own embodied experiences. While it's possible that those accounts are embellished or fraudulent, in order to gain a broader understanding of disability in the Civil War North, we must trust the evidence of soldiers' experience of their own bodies.

A note about word choices and definitions: language can be tricky in disability history. Many of the terms that nineteenth-century Americans used, such as *cripple* and *insane*, are now inappropriate, while the terminology we use today was less common or unknown at the time. In this study, I minimize my use of terms that are no longer preferred today. But in some places, these terms are necessary to demonstrate the mind-set of Civil War–era Americans. I also use my word choice to challenge us to think about the ways that disability functions within a person's life. Rather than describing a soldier as *maimed* or *broken*, I opt for terms like *altered* or *changed* to try to shift the conversation away from how disability *destroyed* men's lives and toward how it *changed* men's lives. Too often, a disabled life is portrayed as one not worth living. Perhaps some of the men who appear in these chapters felt that way, but disabled soldiers and veterans more often experienced the full range of human emotions, feeling joy and pain and boredom and sadness like any typically abled person. While much of this book necessarily dwells on the difficult aspects of living with a wartime disability, I do not intend to portray disabled lives as worthless.

Defining disability is also complicated because what is and is not considered a disability changes over time, varies across region, and is informed by a variety of social, cultural, and environmental factors. A significant point of scholarly debate is whether illness should be considered a disability, particularly because of the work that has been done to shift from the medical model of analysis to the social model. Illness remains the domain of medical professionals and is often curable, and modern scholars generally do not consider it a disability.[12] However, I choose to include illness within my use of the term *disabled* in this book for three reasons. First, disease made it difficult or impossible for men to successfully navigate their environment (camp, the march, and combat) or adhere to codes of military behavior and was thus disabling. Second, the War Department categorized ill health as a disability during the war in that profoundly sick men were discharged as "disabled." Similarly, the Pension Bureau considered the effects of ill health pensionable disabilities. Third, many of the diseases soldiers contracted during the war gave them permanent chronic symptoms or left them susceptible to other infections. For example, Dora Costa finds that malaria increased rates of chronic illness in Union veterans for decades after the war's end.[13] Disability and illness were not (and are not) one and the same, but neither were they mutually exclusive.

Definitions of disability are at the center of the first two chapters. In chapter 1, we consider the Invalid Corps, later renamed the Veteran Reserve Corps, as the institution in which the state first formulated its response to the sick and wounded men the war created. The army faced a twofold problem: a large population of disabled men, and a growing need for manpower in the ranks. In order to maintain troop strength, the War Department created the corps as a place where men deemed unfit for field service could still perform useful and necessary tasks. However, the anxieties that the disabled soldier's body inspired were embedded within the Invalid Corps's creation. In addition to its practical purpose, the Invalid Corps strove to save disabled men from becoming dependent paupers. But as this chapter explores, many soldiers believed that rather than saving them, the unit separated and stigmatized them as unfit. Defining disability, and determining who had the power over those definitions, was a central tension. Soldiers chafed at being labeled unfit and longed for their old units, and disparities between the ailments of enlisted men and officers revealed the beginnings of a hierarchy of disability.

On the other side of the coin, chapter 2 focuses on the experiences of soldiers that I refer to as the "walking sick." These men testified to being impaired, but not enough so for their superiors to consider them disabled. Just as soldiers, surgeons, and officers remained conflicted over what impairments warranted a soldier's transfer to the Invalid Corps, they disagreed about how severe an impairment had to be before a soldier earned accommodation in the form of hospitalization or extra rest. Despite their condition, the men of the Invalid Corps wished to avoid categorization as disabled. Conversely, the walking sick actively sought that designation because it might afford them benefits like medical care, rest, or discharge. These conflicts amounted to more than just grumbling in the ranks. This chapter uses court-martial records as a window into the tensions between military masculinity, disability, and power for the walking wounded.

Disabled soldiers' and veterans' bodies helped create the meanings and memory of the war. Examination of the ways in which this meaning was constructed is an important thread running throughout Civil War disability scholarship. Many recent histories of disabled veterans focus on war wounds' symbolic use in postwar discussions of reconciliation and memory creation.[14] This thread appears here, too, though in a more literal sense. The first two chapters of this study demonstrate disabled bodies' usefulness in maintaining the fighting strength of the Union army.

On an even more literal level, chapter 3 emphasizes disabled bodies' utility for medical research. As Dr. Sartorius takes ownership of Albion Simms as a token of medical fascination, the doctors of the Army Medical Department used body parts of wounded and dead soldiers to help advance medical science. Because they had the authority to label a soldier disabled while in the ranks, surgeons and officers held immense power over their patients' bodies. They used that authority to fill the shelves of the newly created Army Medical Museum with specimens to aid in the education of future American physicians. The museum's curators tried to frame the collection of white soldiers' body parts as an extension of their patriotic duty as citizen-soldiers. But the bones were displayed alongside remains gathered for their racial and physical otherness, undermining the argument that disabled soldiers and veterans were privileged among marginalized groups.

The Army Medical Museum also made war wounds highly visible. Visitors could see shattered skulls and amputated limbs firsthand and ponder the role such wounds played in the conflict. Put more succinctly, the museum and its exhibits offered visitors the opportunity to stare. The case of Joshua Lawrence Chamberlain, explored in chapter 4, shows just how much both the state and the public desired to better understand war wounds, and struggled to understand those injuries not easily seen. Chamberlain received a severe wound through the hips that changed his life in significant ways, but he is almost never understood as disabled because his wounds were concealed under his clothing. Moreover, he had a fairly typical life after the war. By exploring Chamberlain's life with the wound and his experiences with the Pension Bureau, this chapter suggests that nonvisible disabilities complicate our ideas about war wounds as patriotic sacrifices, as well as the assumption that disabled lives are by necessity bitter and miserable.

Building on that discussion of the Pension Bureau, chapter 5 shifts our focus to the postwar era to examine the delicate maneuvers disabled Civil War veterans undertook to receive pensions. While it is true that an enormous number of veterans were pensioned by the turn of the century, the process was far from a simple ask and ye shall receive. Not only did old soldiers have to navigate a sea of paperwork, they also had to describe their ailments in ways that fit the Pension Bureau's definition of pensionable disability. Many Americans resented the growing pension rolls but had to be careful not to criticize men considered the saviors of the Union. This chapter demonstrates that bureaucrats, aided by the partisan press, developed the work-around of using gendered moral grounds to separate worthy veterans from the unworthy. Former soldiers were evaluated based on their manhood—men who exhibited bad moral fiber, seemed like whiners, or failed to bear their pain with appropriate stoicism could all be relegated to the ranks of the unworthy. Veterans' worth became more than a theoretical discussion in the pages of newspapers, however, when Pres. Grover Cleveland began vetoing individual pension bills, calling out the failings of the veterans seeking support.

In the final chapter, we turn to mental illness—the least visible of all Civil War disabilities, the most difficult to understand for those who lived with it, and the one that has caused perhaps the most debate among historians. Using the patient case files of three institutions along with the letters of inmates and their families, chapter 6 meditates on how former Union soldiers and their families experienced war trauma and institutionalization. In each case, patients, families, or physicians identified the war as having played a role in the mental disability. Thus the chapter is less an examination of whether war trauma existed and more a close reading of the way some postwar Americans experienced it. These documents make clear that war-related mental illness was individual as well as relational. Soldiers grappled with the emasculating stigma of the asylum while their symptoms and institutionalization strained, and in many cases tore, family bonds. For these soldiers and their families, the separation and heartache of the war did not end in 1865. For some, it did not end at all.

So we begin our journey into the bodily toll the Civil War exacted, but rather than assuming the viewpoint of Dr. Sartorius, fascinated by the medical miracle, we will take the perspective of men like Albion Simms. The bodies of disabled Union soldiers and veterans were sites of powerful cultural beliefs about duty, honor, and sacrifice. Yet those ideals could transform into weapons to be used against men who failed to properly perform the role of wounded warrior. Under the gaze of surgeons, officers, bureaucrats, and civilians, disabled soldiers made difficult negotiations in their attempts to accommodate impaired bodies. Some managed this process with ease; others floundered, struggled, and suffered. All of it, the light and the dark, is the history of Civil War disability.

CHAPTER 1

Gather the Invalids

On December 13, 1862, the Fifth New Hampshire, part of Winfield Scott Hancock's Second Corps, advanced up Marye's Heights to attack James Longstreet's Confederate corps. The battle was intense; barrage of shot and shell hammered the regiment. Col. Edward Cross recalled in his diary that the casualties were so heavy, it seemed as though "men fell like grass before the scythe."[1] By the end of the day, 180 of the 249 New Hampshire men were dead or wounded. Among the casualties was twenty-two-year-old regimental musician George Farnum. He had been, in his own words, "with the rest of the cattle" as they "were driven into the jaws of death before the death-dealing batteries on the heights beyond the city of Fredericksburg."[2] Farnum felt a "smart blow" to his right shoulder and assumed he had collided with a comrade in the chaos. Soon, though, he felt warm blood running down his arm. The blow had actually been a gunshot to the shoulder; his arm dangled, unresponsive, at his side.

Farnum headed for the rear, where the surgeon decided his wound was too severe to be treated in camp. He was then transferred to the New Hallowell Hospital in Alexandria, Virginia, to recuperate. Farnum chafed at being kept cooped up, and though Alexandria offered amusing diversions for a "hospital bummer," he just wanted to get back to his regiment. The examining medical director had other plans. In November, Farnum was transferred to the newly formed Invalid Corps.[3] He was not pleased: "Here I am, an unwilling member of the corps, denominated in Washington, 'The United States Paupers.'"[4]

The Invalid Corps, later renamed the Veteran Reserve Corps (VRC), was formed in the spring of 1863 as a reserve unit for sick and disabled soldiers.

Though its official purpose was maintaining troop strength, the corps also functioned as a crucible in which the Union army shaped its definition of disability and began forming its response to the bodily crisis of the Civil War. Bodies were necessary to keeping the war machine running smoothly. As the ranks thinned in the second and third years of the war, it seemed foolish to simply discharge the sick or wounded. The War Department had the power to decide what it meant to be a disabled soldier, and to determine what tasks disabled men could perform so that no potential labor was lost. Many believed that by keeping these soldiers in the ranks performing meaningful war work, the Invalid Corps might also spare them the emasculation of relying on pensions. But soldiers resented performing tasks associated with women, free blacks, and contraband slaves. Members of the Invalid Corps found themselves in the awkward space between soldier and invalid, where they were categorized simultaneously as able and unable. In turn, they were both honored and lampooned. Foreshadowing later developments in the veteran pension system, the Invalid Corps revealed the complicated and sometimes contradictory ways that state, society, and soldier interpreted wartime disability.

The Civil War presented, as LeeAnn Whites famously states, a crisis in gender.[5] The men who populated the Union army came from various cultures across the North, bringing with them unique ideas about what it meant to be a white man. Differing notions about manhood created tension and conflict, but the war also offered shared gendered experiences.[6] For some, the crisis stemmed from the expectation and social pressure to serve. Others perceived the war as a test of their manhood, either confirming their capabilities or revealing their weakness and cowardice.[7] For nearly all of the men who fought in the Union army, the war presented one other gendered crisis—a sick or wounded body.

Nineteenth-century Americans associated disability with dependency and emasculation. Independence and self-sufficiency were vital aspects of both manhood and citizenship dating back to the Revolutionary era, but these required physical and mental ability.[8] While economic production was centered in the home, early American disabled veterans avoided dependency because families shared required household labor, and disabled family members participated in the capacity they were able.[9] When wage earning became the standard during the market revolution, those unable to achieve economic independence became dependent on wage-earning white men. Some considered this dependency natural: women and children, for example, could not be economically independent and relied on male heads of household to care and provide for them. Black Americans were also deemed biologically incapable of true independence, and even free blacks were often considered dependent members of white households.[10] White men held positions of both power and responsibility, as they were expected to provide for dependents. Those who failed to fulfill that role and instead lived on support from the state or their neighbors were considered degraded paupers.[11]

During the Civil War, a battle wound could potentially upend this hierarchy, preventing white men from providing for their families and making them rely on wives, children, and attendants. Of course, such traumas, imbued with beliefs about patriotic and manful sacrifice, differed from the typical antebellum disabilities. War wounds, especially obvious ones like amputations, carried a certain amount of social capital in a society eager to celebrate the sacrifices of brave citizen-soldiers. As Frances Clarke shows, civilians praised amputees as exemplars of the citizen-soldier ideal.[12] Yet patriotic sacrifice or no, war wounds challenged central tenets of manhood. Injuries altered male bodies and raised concerns about men's ability to attract mates, father children, support families, or remain independent. While notions of mid-nineteenth-century masculinity were diverse, self-control remained a powerful common element of manhood in all its various incarnations. Genteel middle-class men should control physical indulgences or outbursts, while working-class men believed self-control included the manipulation and use of their bodies in fighting or physical feats. Importantly, each definition of masculine self-control hinged on the right and ability to control one's own body.[13] Even when wounded or disabled, soldiers and veterans were expected to act, speak, and move as if the disability did not exist.[14]

Self-control also marked a critical difference between white and black bodies, as enslaved and freed men had no control over their physical integrity and were precluded from using their bodies in the same ways as white men. Black men were often at the mercy of the overseer's whip or the master's financial whims. Further, racism and slavery barred black men from activities white men believed earned honor, such as dueling, fighting, or feats of physical prowess. Indeed, the right to endanger their bodies in military service has often been interpreted as a watershed moment when former slaves and free blacks became men in the eyes of whites.[15] To be unable to control one's own body, whether for physiological or ideological reasons, was to assume the place not only of a dependent, but also of someone who lacked the basic powers of manhood. For disabled soldiers, even if they had less control over their physical functions, continued service in their own regiments might at least allow them to project able-bodiedness. Separated, issued unique uniforms, and labeled unfit, members of the Invalid Corps found themselves in the one place where they could not pretend.

The Invalid Corps resulted from a desire to formalize disabled soldiers' labor and maximize the Union army's troop strength and efficiency. Manpower was a legitimate concern in 1863, when the federal government was growing increasingly anxious that the army was shrinking. The North had a larger male population of military age and, in the end, a much larger army than the Confederacy. However, Paul Cimbala notes that the Union army had significant responsibilities beyond the front lines, such as defense of the capital, the imperialistic conquest of Native Americans in the West, and various other duties.[16] That spring, the War Department took steps to increase troop strength through enlistment. In March, President Lincoln had signed the Enrollment Act authorizing a draft on all Northern men between the ages of twenty and forty-five. The War Department's General Order 143, released in late May, authorized the enlistment of black men into the ranks and established the United States Colored Troops. As the War Department actively sought new populations from which to draw soldiers, many began to question the protocols regarding the convalescence and discharge of sick and wounded men.

Typically, when a soldier was hurt or sick while serving in the field, his first stop was the regimental surgeon. Ideally, the medical problem could be handled within the soldier's own unit so that he could quickly return to service. If his ailment was severe, however, remaining with his regiment would hinder its mobility. Troops requiring a longer recovery time or more intensive medical treatment were transferred to division or general hospitals. This move meant that soldiers could receive more specialized care and better rest. It also meant that large populations of men past the critical stages of their conditions but still too sick to return to field service remained in the hospital, taking up beds, using supplies, and sometimes getting into trouble. As a result, many surgeons found it easier to offer furloughs to men healthy enough to travel and recuperate at home.[17] Other doctors, whether hoping to rid themselves of troublesome patients or reward their favorites, opted to simply discharge soldiers.

Surgeons, then, were on the front lines of a looming manpower crisis. Indeed, their role proved so critical that army surgeon Roberts Bartholow stated that "giving a certificate of disability for discharge is one of the most important duties a military surgeon has to perform."[18] In the earliest years of the war, a lack of strict guidance on qualifications for a disability discharge left surgeons with a great deal of discretion and the army with a seemingly unnecessary number of released soldiers. According to Bartholow, by May 1863, 143,303 men had been discharged on certificates of disability. However, he guessed that a more accurate total would be closer to 200,000.[19]

In order to stave off a manpower shortage, the army would have to staunch the exodus of convalescents and better control their labor once they were retained. The perception that hospitals were full of soldiers who were more or less healthy but technically still recovering was not unwarranted. Explaining, "Soldiers must go somewhere to kill time," George Farnum described bored recuperating men frequenting the circus and theater and enjoying parties.[20] Margaret Humphreys's analysis of Satterlee Hospital in Philadelphia shows that patients drank and caroused, played billiards and cards, attended lectures and other entertainments, causing some to assume that many were "shammers."[21] Of course, sickness and disability and having fun were not mutually exclusive. In fact, entertainment was part of the treatment plan for soldiers at Satterlee. Surgeons believed that idleness bred morale problems, and activity—even in the pursuit of pleasure—helped soldiers heal.

Work also constituted a way of keeping active, and surgeons frequently required that soldiers perform tasks around the hospital. Disabled and convalescent soldiers had been used as informal hospital workers since the start of the war; they were often expected to pitch in while they recuperated. In April 1862, the War Department's General Order 36 attempted to make soldiers' ad hoc hospital work into a more official arrangement, authorizing the chief medical officer of each city to employ as "nurses, cooks, and attendants any convalescent, wounded, or feeble men" who could work, rather than discharging them.[22] Though intended to better manage convalescents' labor, the order was vague and could hardly be characterized as strict. It was also not clear whether recovering soldiers should be discharged or retained. Just days before, Edwin Stanton had ordered medical officers to discharge all soldiers who would be unfit for duty for at least thirty days if they so requested.[23] Though some did stay, many soldiers certainly would have preferred resting at home to performing drudge work around a government hospital. Roberts Bartholow bemoaned General Order 36, complaining, "This regulation, from causes which it is not necessary at this time to relate, proved to be inapplicable, and was practically ignored."[24]

Even when the order functioned as intended and soldiers continued to work, the system remained disorganized. No mechanism existed for tracking how long these soldiers had been on light duty or when they should be returned to the ranks. Additionally, rather than answering to a military chain of command, soldiers reported only to surgeons. This weak oversight made it easier for some men to take advantage of the system, biding their time in the safety of the hospital rather than returning to the front, or getting discharged by a surgeon happy to be rid of them. Such soldiers were labeled "bummers" and considered akin to malingerers—immoral cowards desperate to avoid a fight.[25] A newspaper article criticizing antiwar factions after Appomattox lumped in bummers with other despised groups, claiming that the Democratic Party in one Pennsylvania town was "made up of negro buyers, negro sellers, negro drivers, secessionists, deserters, Canada skedaddlers, Western skedaddlers, skulkers, hospital bummers, guerrillas, bushwackers, barn-burners, amnestied rebels, rebel sympathizers, Knights of the Golden Circle, Sons of Liberty, and spies."[26] It also continued to be relatively simple for convalescent soldiers to sneak away on unauthorized leave. When Alfred Bellard grew restless while recuperating from a leg wound in the hospital during the summer of 1863, he took it on himself to go home for a month.[27]

Straggling or deserted soldiers sometimes took refuge among those who had been ordered to the hospital, hoping to blend in and avoid returning to the front. In George Farnum's opinion, fault lay with surgeons who kept their favorite soldiers in the safety and ease of the infirmary. After a supervising medical officer inspected patients at New Hallowell in the summer of 1863, Farnum reported several doctors' displeasure that their evaluation of their own patients would be superseded: "Most of them were ordered to report to their respective regiments for duty, as they were able-bodied men, but were favorites of the surgeons and were reported as unfit for field service, in order to retain them here."[28] The presence of even a few shirkers cast doubt on all convalescing soldiers, particularly when they were working around the hospital or taking in the entertainments of the city. Even if the pastimes were lifting spirits and shortening recovery times, many deemed them incompatible with true sickness. Moreover, these pursuits reinforced the idea that large numbers of the patients in hospitals and convalescent camps were shirkers.

Concern arose that soldiers might be very good—perhaps even too good—at hospital work. The Sanitary Commission believed that convalescent soldiers were "most satisfactory" compared to sometimes overzealous volunteers because they were more accustomed to discipline and authority.[29] Although War Department officials acknowledged that disabled troops' labor was useful, they also believed that hospital service might eat away at the men's identity as soldiers. Both women and men performed these tasks, but male hospital workers were typically black or disabled.[30] Nursing, cooking, or otherwise doing relief work positioned white soldiers in the role of those considered incapable of the "real" work of war. It seemed a logical conclusion that these types of duties would ruin them for soldiering. "The invalids thus occupied were useful indeed," John W. DeForest recalled, "but they ceased to be soldiers in fact and spirit."[31] Whether convalescing soldiers were useful or not, performing hospital labor could potentially chip away at their soldierly manhood, leaving them unprepared to return to the hardships of life on the front lines.

March 1863 marked another attempt to organize disabled hospital laborers when the War Department required these soldiers answer to a more formal chain of command consisting of officers rather than surgeons.[32] While this policy change clarified the command hierarchy, it failed to solve all the difficulties of using convalescing soldiers as hospital workers. Soldiers often remained on the rolls of their regiments but were not present for duty, falsely inflating troop strength. As Paul Cimbala writes, "The men continued to perform services in and around the military hospitals, but the arrangements still remained ad hoc, temporary, and without an overarching military rationale."[33] Unable to keep large numbers of recuperating men at hospitals, surgeons discharged many who were disabled only "for the march and bivouac" but "entirely competent to act as garrison troops and provost-police."[34]

The Invalid Corps therefore came to fruition in April 1863 under Secretary of War Edwin Stanton's General Order 105.[35] In his official report on the history of the organization, John W. DeForest, adjutant general of the Invalid Corps, explained that this step "sprang from a national necessity. So severe was the draft of the war on the able-bodied manhood of the American people that an intelligent economy of the public forces demanded that some portion of the vast number of men ... unfit for field service should be utilized for military purposes." It only made sense to "keep in service experienced soldiers who were simply disabled for the march." Rather than waiting long periods of time for these men to fully recover in the hospital, the military would put them to work as soon as they were out of immediate risk.[36]

From this point onward, disability discharges were reserved for men who had undergone an amputation (though they could choose transfer to the Invalid Corps), men with certain severe infirmities, and men whose recovery time outweighed the time left on their enlistment. Otherwise, the order forbade the discharge of any man fitting the criteria for service in the Invalid Corps. Further, General Order 212, which outlined the specific regulations for the corps, required that all soldiers in general hospitals and convalescent camps "perform such hospital or military duty" as they were able until a medical officer could determine whether they belonged in the ranks or the Invalid Corps, or whether they required a discharge.[37] Instead of an ad hoc system in which they were chosen to perform hospital work, disabled soldiers now faced a mandate to work as soon as they were deemed sufficiently fit.

The Invalid Corps helped to remedy inefficient use of convalescent labor, but it also recast the way Americans thought about wartime disability. Receiving a battle wound or becoming ill no longer constituted the culmination of a soldier's obligation to the army. Rather, these events marked the start of a renewed duty. In order to fill the ranks of the newly organized corps, the War Department had to determine what it meant to be disabled, which meant parsing the endless possibilities of wartime ailments and their effects. For instance, what degree of diarrheal illness was simply a reality of life in the army, and what degree made it impossible for a soldier to continue serving in the field? General Order 212 outlines criteria for myriad ailments and conditions. Roberts Bartholow's *Manual of Instructions for Enlisting and Discharging Soldiers* details these standards. Drafted at the urging of Surgeon General William A. Hammond, Bartholow's work was designed for Army Medical Department distribution to surgeons in the field. The Invalid Corps necessitated a new definition of disability requiring that men be declared unfit for field service but fit for certain tasks. Thus, labor and productivity defined disability. The War Department interpreted disability as a continuum of degrees rather than a state of being—incapacitated or able-bodied.[38]

Most obvious illnesses, chronic conditions, and injuries warranted inclusion in the Invalid Corps. General Order 212 listed the "physical infirmities" that made soldiers incapable of field service, but did "not disqualify them for service in the Invalid Corps." These included some ailments that seemed fairly serious, such as epilepsy, chronic diarrhea or pain, and the loss of part or all of a limb. The key to properly determining a soldier's status, Roberts Bartholow counseled his fellow surgeons, was carefully assessing the degree of a disability. For example, while epilepsy did not disqualify a soldier for the Invalid Corps, a more severe case—more than one seizure a month—did. Degree was particularly important when it came to conditions like chronic diarrhea, which led to thousands of discharges each year. While some men were too weak to continue to be of use, many could certainly still serve as a clerk or garrison guard.

Bartholow carefully parsed even gunshot wounds. "Wounds of the chest, not implicating organs, do not disqualify for service in the invalid battalions," he wrote. If one was unlucky enough to have a wound implicating the lungs, it would "disqualify [him] for field service and for the first battalion . . . but not for the second, unless followed by collapse of lung, empyema, or similar important lesions." A loss of both testes was disqualifying for field service, but not the Invalid Corps; the loss of more than half of the penis, however, warranted a discharge.[39] A separate category of conditions would not be accepted even in the Invalid Corps: "manifest imbecility or insanity," uncontrolled syphilis, "great injuries or diseases of the skull," total blindness and deafness, an artificial anus, or a urinary fistula. These ailments, among others, disqualified soldiers largely because they impacted the men's ability to meet hygiene codes or perform useful work.[40]

The composition of the corps offers some insight into the way the army stratified ailments. Enlisted men were incapacitated largely by disease, reflecting the causes of disability in the army at large. According to *The Medical and Surgical History of the War of the Rebellion*, illness disabled almost three-quarters of the men who entered the Invalid Corps in 1863, and the most common reported ailments were chronic diarrhea and general debility. Just 32 percent of the unit's troops carried battle wounds.[41] The officer corps was more carefully curated. Evaluating boards quizzed potential officers on tactics, regulations, and the Articles of War. Board members also scrutinized candidates' record of service, level of education, and reputation for discipline and sobriety. This process ensured that only the most deserving received commissions—partly in a preemptive strike against those who might accuse the corps of being a repository for both the infirm and inferior.[42]

Further, the Provost Marshal General's Office, in charge of commissioning officers for the corps, favored men wounded in battle over men suffering from disease.[43] Of the 427 men commissioned into the Invalid Corps as officers, 389 (89 percent) had been physically wounded. Of that number, 77 (18 percent) had undergone an amputation. Just 39 (9.1 percent) were disabled only by illness: 8 from chronic diarrhea, 5 from rheumatism, 5 for hernias, and the rest for various ailments ranging from phthisis to kidney disease.[44] As a result, it was difficult for those in the field service to accuse the officers of the Invalid Corps of being shirkers seeking out the easier path—their bodies bore proof of their dedication to the cause.

War wounds might have spoken to soldiers' valor, but they also meant that the resulting officer corps was a veritable encyclopedia of the things war would do to the human body. Robert E. Johnston, a young soldier from West Virginia who became a lieutenant colonel in the Invalid Corps, "received wounds from musket balls in [the] mouth and neck, and in the left shoulder from shell."[45] First Lt. Louis Ahrens was shot in both legs and the right arm, while First Lt. C. S. Schaeffer was shot in the head and received a shell wound to the spine.[46] Capt. William Brian was wounded, taken prisoner, released, then wounded and taken prisoner again, all between 1861 and the end of 1862. Ultimately, he had been "wounded in [the] right leg, in the left breast, in the right hip, and had his left leg amputated while prisoner ... in Libby prison."[47] Enlisted men, on the other hand, overwhelmingly wound up in the corps for altogether less glorious reasons like diarrhea and debility, reinforcing the commonly held belief that wounded soldiers were better and braver than those who suffered from camp illnesses.

The categories of disability implemented by the Invalid Corps rested on the foundation of mid-nineteenth-century beliefs about manhood, labor, and productivity. Concerns arose early in the war over what would become of sick and wounded soldiers when they were discharged. According to Provost Marshal General James B. Fry, one of the express purposes of the Invalid Corps was preventing soldiers' dependency on their families and communities. In his 1863 report to Secretary of War Edwin Stanton, Fry identified the Invalid Corps's two objectives. The first, of course, was to retain disabled soldiers and officers within the army to perform important but light military duties. Second, the corps was to "provide honorable and useful occupation and suitable compensation for a class of persons whose claims upon the nation no one can question." The Invalid Corps, then, was founded not only to help maintain troop strength, but also to ensure disabled soldiers' employment. "Men who have become disabled in the military service of the country are thus supported by the Government," Fry wrote, "they ... strengthen the active armies, and, though more or less disabled, they earn, and have the satisfaction of feeling that they earn, the compensation bestowed upon them."[48]

The government supported disabled soldiers by ensuring their continued service in the Invalid Corps. But duty in the corps also meant that ailing soldiers continued to labor for the army while the government avoided paying pensions. Fry noted, "[By serving in this] corps of honor the pride and soldierly spirit which produced their battle scars is fostered and protected by giving them useful and honorable employment, instead of leaving them inactive and in want, a burden to themselves and to the community."[49] The 1862 Act to Grant Pensions offered a government pension to each Union soldier disabled during his time in the army. But from the beginning, the act placed soldiers in a difficult position. Though pensions were fashioned so that the nation could repay its debt to soldiers who had sacrificed for the Union, men who accepted pensions became passive recipients of government support. In other words, they became dependents. Even though the pension system was created to prevent this status, Fry's letter suggests that the idea of adult men relying on the government for support still carried a stigma, even when cast as a debt owed by a grateful nation. War wounds may have been praised as the ultimate proof of manhood, but they were not quite enough to prove a soldier's masculinity. Even the battle-scarred, it was feared, risked joining the ranks of the undeserving poor.

The Invalid Corps, however, offered an ideal solution to this problem. Soldiers received "adequate pay, clothing, and subsistence," and they avoided being "mere recipients of a public charity."[50] The corps, then, became more than a way to preserve manpower; the War Department saw it as way for disabled soldiers to preserve their manhood. At the same time, the corps also offered a considerable financial advantage for the Union army and the federal government. Soldiers transferred to the Invalid Corps could not receive pensions while in the service, and they were ineligible for bounties or premiums. Moreover, they continued to receive the same rate of pay as the rest of the army. If discharged, these soldiers would be able to draw their pensions, which the government paid out with no labor offered in return. Their absence would need to be offset by another soldier's labor, at the very least nearly doubling the expense for the government.[51]

Those on the home front shared the idea that the Invalid Corps served a greater purpose than bolstering troop strength. According to some interpretations, the unit's primary aim was saving soldiers from pauperism. "The great object of this Corps is to give honorable employment to those who have lost health or limbs in the service, and are unfit for other employments," reported the editors of the Amherst, New Hampshire, *Farmer's Cabinet*.[52] A Maryland newspaper called the Invalid Corps a long-awaited answer to the question, "What provision does the Government intend to make for its disabled soldiers?" Finally, the writer stated, "the maimed and enfeebled soldier is provided for, and the citizen is no longer deterred from enlisting in the army, for fear of beggary, should the fortune of war deprive him of the means of support by his labor." Those who had already been wounded in the war "were not to be cast upon the charity of the world as no longer of value."[53]

The *New York Evening Post* suggested that the disabled men entering the Invalid Corps should be thankful that the government was offering them an opportunity be "placed in every respect on an equality with all other soldiers." A soldier in the corps could feel "pride and satisfaction" that he was earning his pay rather than receiving a pension. The creation of the Invalid Corps shaped a definition of disability that reinforced the cultural connection between disability and labor and the conflict between manhood and dependency. That definition would have lasting repercussions in the postwar era. Pensions were just beginning to influence ideas about manhood and disability, but the Invalid Corps offered an escape valve for any serious debate over their payment. That opportunity for escape would no longer exist after Appomattox.

The rank and file of the Invalid Corps were organized into two battalions. Those "most efficient and able-bodied, and capable of using the musket, and performing guard duty, light marches, &c." formed First Battalion. Second Battalion contained "those of the next degree of physical efficiency, including those who [had] lost a hand or an arm." An additional proposed battalion, which would include those who had lost a leg or foot and were thus deemed "least effective," never materialized. Therefore, men with lower limb amputations joined the Second Battalion.[54] The ranks filled in fairly quickly, and by the fall of 1863 the new organization comprised 16 regiments, 203 companies, and 18,255 men.[55] First Battalion, consisting of comparatively healthier soldiers, was always significantly larger than its counterpart. In fact, many members of the Second Battalion found that their health improved, likely due to the chance for rest and easy access to medical care, after a few months' service. These men were often transferred into the First Battalion as they got healthier.

Both battalions served the provost marshal, but the soldiers' state of health dictated their function. The soldiers of First Battalion, generally less severely wounded or sick, served a variety of functions, acting as escorts for new troops, prison guards, and garrison pickets. In addition, these men served as military police, particularly on the home front. Members of First Battalion were allowed to carry rifles, and they were more likely to be involved in unexpected scrapes, especially when monitoring the draft or guarding prisoners. Some First Battalion soldiers skirmished with Rebels at Fort Stevens in 1864, for example. Others were injured—and one died—in clashes with protesters during the 1863 New York City draft riots. Service in the Invalid Corps did not necessarily mean a life of leisure, especially in First Battalion. Alfred Bellard, shot in the knee at Chancellorsville, served as a military police officer and prison guard in Washington, DC, and he recalled in his memoir how very physical his job could be. On more than one occasion, Bellard restrained angry prisoners or carried drunken soldiers back to their barracks.[56] Second Battalion was less likely to encounter such situations. Considered less capable because of their missing limbs, the unit's men carried swords and handguns rather than long guns, and they served mostly within hospital settings, working as orderlies, cooks, and nurses. Some of these soldiers labored as clerks or supply workers.[57] Though necessary for the support and efficiency of the Union army, this work was a far cry from the military experience that most soldiers had come to know, and, in spite of the grind, toil, and terror, often missed.

Medical transfers made up the vast majority of the soldiers in the Invalid Corps. Indeed, most of those who entered the ranks were like George Farnum—men who had no choice but to be transferred.[58] Farnum had hoped to get back to his regiment, and he had gone so far as to elicit a promise from the surgeon at the New Hallowell Hospital in Alexandria that he would be returned. But the medical director—the surgeon's superior—had overridden the pledge and relegated Farnum to the Invalid Corps. Certainly, after his service with the Fifth New Hampshire, well-known throughout the army as a seasoned regiment with a storied if bloody history, joining a unit that would brand each of its members an "invalid" was disappointing.

Farnum, who had been writing to the Amherst, New Hampshire, newspaper the *Farmer's Cabinet* under the alias "A Member of the N.H. Fifth Regiment," made no attempt to mask his frustration. He submitted his bitter November 1863 letter from an "Ex-Member of the N.H. Fifth Regiment," and though he had typically signed his other correspondence "G. H. F.," he identified himself only as "Invalid." Farnum's transfer put him in a black mood. "It was more anger than grief or low spirits," he wrote, "attended with disgust and a little shame at being forced into Uncle Sam's Almhouse."[59] His snarky references to the corps as an almshouse, the "United States Paupers," and the "cripple corps" revealed the real ambivalence some disabled soldiers felt toward the unit. Being wounded in the line of duty, though it meant living with the pain and stigma of disability, also offered a certain amount of social capital. A soldier with a wound such as Farnum's—serious but healed, and not life-threatening—would certainly have received some honors both in the field and at home. But rather than receive either, he remained in a kind of limbo, segregated with other sick and wounded men, kept from the front lines, and labeled an "invalid." For Farnum, his new status only reinforced the idea that disabled soldiers were damaged goods.

Farnum was certainly not alone in his frustration with his transfer to the Invalid Corps. Walter Dunn, a teenaged private in the Eleventh New Jersey, was shot in the throat at Chancellorsville. The ball passed through his lung and lodged in his shoulder, causing respiratory problems, motion impairment, and pain. Dunn experienced numerous setbacks in his recovery from the severe wound. The ball moved within his shoulder, and his lung became infected, confining him to Baltimore's Jarvis Hospital for months. Tired of all the rest, Dunn began to volunteer as a nurse around Jarvis while he waited for clearance to return to the field. In October, Dunn learned that instead of going back to his unit, he would be transferred to the Second Battalion of the Invalid Corps. The thought made him wistful: "As soon as I am mustered in the I.C. I have nothing more to do with the 11th Regiment of NJ or that with me, my name is then crossed off all company books."[60]

When a rumor circulated that Second Battalion was going to be dissolved and its soldiers either folded into First Battalion or discharged, Dunn insisted he would not be transferred into another unit of the Invalid Corps: "Either my regiment or a discharge, no 1st Battalion I.C. for me, no, no." He longed for both the dangers and glories of the front. "I am quite tired of this inactive life," he complained. "I prefer one of action and am soon going to do what I can to be transferred back to the Bloody 11th and share with my comrades the fate of war."[61] After the surrender, he hoped he might somehow travel back to New Jersey with the old Eleventh and muster out with the unit—though he was no longer a member.[62]

Walter Dunn's longing for the old Eleventh showed how service in the Invalid Corps disrupted the powerful bonds of regimental comradeship. The fact that some soldiers wanted reassignment to field service seems to have been a well-known criticism of the corps. As John W. DeForest reported, "Men frequently begged to be sent back to their old regiments in the field rather than remain in garrison at the price of being called invalids."[63] In January 1865, a New York *World* editorial argued that disabled soldiers disliked being removed from beloved comrades and regiments: "Ask the first maimed soldier, with a hospital pass in his pocket, whom you may meet in the street, whether he desires his transfer to the Veteran Reserve Corps and he will tell you with a sneer, 'No! Let me have my discharge, or be sent back to my regiment.'" The writer attributed this attitude to the practice of drawing regiments from neighborhoods, which gave soldiers a sense of kinship with their comrades.[64] The Invalid Corps took soldiers away from this community to be "transferred to a heterogeneous corps composed of representatives of all states and nations."[65] The men understood that they had something in common with their new comrades. But rather than being part of the "Bloody 11th" and sharing in their regiment's honors, they were now identified primarily by their disability. For many soldiers, assignment to the Invalid Corps stripped them of the identities they had cultivated while serving with their units.

The Invalid Corps's uniform reinforced the sense that its soldiers were being segregated from the rest of the army. The unit was assigned its own uniform of "dark-blue forage cap and sky-blue trousers . . . and a sky-blue kersey jacket, trimmed with dark blue and cut long in the waist."[66] The different color pattern differentiated Invalid Corps soldiers from those in the active service so that disabled men behind the front lines would not be suspected of shirking or straggling. Yet this distinction offended members of the corps, who believed they had earned a right to their dark-blue active service uniforms, and disliked being so obviously marked as a member of the Invalid Corps. Soldiers' attachment to their regulation blue garments was more than preference. As Joseph Beilein notes, the sameness of military uniforms helped to create and reinforce bonds between men, to emphasize their literal uniformity.[67] Disabled soldiers—often already disrupting the sameness with their physical differences—could no longer participate in this visual comradeship.

Able-bodied soldiers also noted the uniform difference, associating it with the belief that the Invalid Corps was second-rate. "Some of the Colonels &c did not like the idea of 'coming into the field to be Commanded by an Invalid,' they did not like the *light blue*," Col. Charles F. Johnson wrote to his wife in June 1864, when several able-bodied regiments came under his command while he was stationed outside Washington, DC. The light-blue uniform became a kind of shorthand for nondisabled troops. This military garb set disabled soldiers apart and confirmed their inferiority in a way that made nondisabled troops resent being commanded by an "Invalid."[68]

Soldiers also took issue with the very name of the organization, which clearly identified its members as lacking in health and ability. Invalids were inactive, passive sufferers sapped of masculine power.[69] Further issues arose when soldiers discovered that the initials of the Invalid Corps—I.C.— were the same as a shorthand the Quartermaster Department used when rejecting supplies. For instance, when they received spoiled meat or shoddy uniforms, quartermasters stamped the crates holding the supplies "I.C.," meaning "Inspected, Condemned." It wasn't long before jokes circulated that members of the Invalid Corps had been "inspected and condemned" themselves. Ninth Corps aide-de-camp Thomas Sturgis recalled how Confederate prisoners under Invalid Corps guard seized on this play on words after the war, referring to their captors as "Condemned Yanks." "The epithet was used so publicly and offensively that these gallant veterans resented the stigma," Sturgis later wrote.[70]

Invalid Corps soldiers sometimes referred to themselves in those terms. Pvt. E. C. Fisk, also medically transferred to the corps, considered the unit "a set of condemned & and in great part useless men."[71] John W. DeForest explained the change in his postwar report by saying that the "bitter prejudice of field troops ... found scope in a multitude of sarcasms and jeers which made the title of Invalid Corps a burden."[72] Embarrassment over the unit's name proved so severe that in March 1864, the Adjutant General's Office

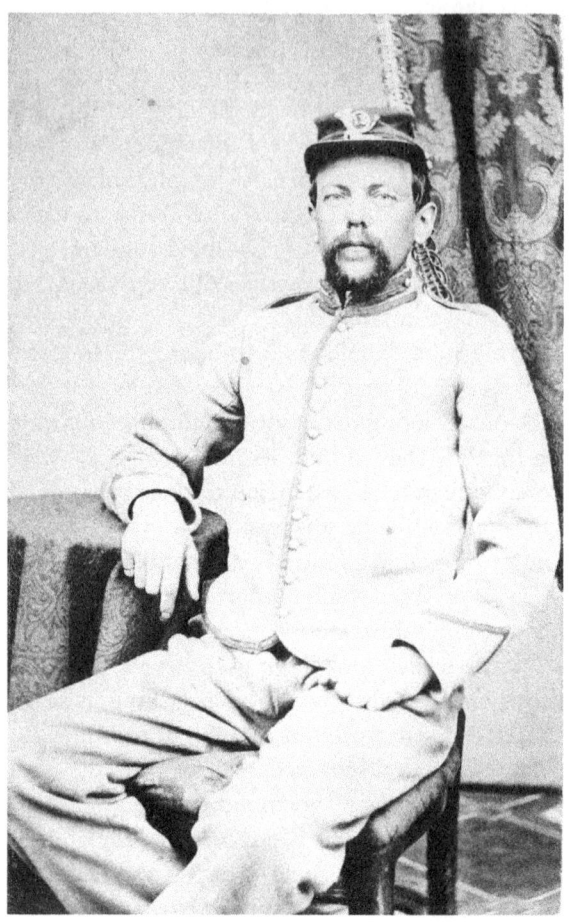

FIGURE 1. Unidentified soldier in Thirteenth Veteran Reserve Corps Infantry Regiment uniform. Photographed by A. K. Josselyn, Gallop's Island, Boston Harbor. Library of Congress Prints and Photographs Division, Washington, DC.

issued General Order 111, officially changing the Invalid Corps's name to the Veteran Reserve Corps. The new designation emphasized not the fitness of soldiers' bodies, but their status as veteran combatants.

James Fry may have wanted the Invalid Corps to be understood primarily as a "corps of honor," but individuals in and out of the army certainly did not interpret it in that way. Popular depictions of the corps contained both mockery and praise. Songs and poetry alternately lauded Invalid Corps soldiers for their honorable scars and accused them of being malingerers and shirkers. Some songwriters' mockery was obvious. In Frank Wilder's popular "The Invalid Corps" (1863), a man who tries to enlist is rejected for his infirmity. The examining surgeon tells the would-be soldier,

> Your lungs are much affected
> And likewise both your eyes are cock'd
> And otherwise defected.

In the chorus, the soldier declares,

> So, now I'm with the Invalids
> And cannot go and fight sir!

Among his new comrades are a man who is too obese, one who is too tall, and one who is too short. The final stanza sums up what the new Invalid Corps looked like:

> Some had the ticerdolerreou
> some what they call "brown critters,"
> and some were "lank and lazy" too,
> Some were too "fond of bitters."
> Some had "cork legs" and some "one eye,"
> with backs deformed and crooked,
> I'll bet you'd laugh'd til you had cried,
> to see how "cute" they looked.[73]

This song's version of the corps *is* populated with rejects, drunks, and fools, not brave wounded soldiers.

The notion of the Invalid Corps as a repository for lousy, immoral soldiers proved pervasive. Critics of the unit suggested that its entry requirements had been made stricter because it was flooded with men who couldn't hack it in the ranks. Specifically, they believed the corps was a haven for men who faked ailments to escape the front lines. Indeed, the attempt to avoid accusations that the Invalid Corps was a refuge for lazy, cowardly, or poor soldiers accounted for tightening guidelines for officer commissions. Yet the allegations did not seem to end. The soldiers of the Invalid Corps, complained one editorialist, "bore too much the reputation of malingerers and skulkers in hospitals, and possessors of weak backs and knees, with remarkable alacrity in falling to the rear at the commencement of trouble, to render association with them at all desirable."[74] The lyrics of "The Invalid Corps" also suggest soldiers were "fond of bitters"—in other words, drunkards. Another song of the same name revolves around a character relegated to the corps after losing an eye. This man drinks with such dedication that he is eventually drummed out.[75]

The above lyrics exploit cultural ideas about both disability and the Invalid Corps for laughs, but the illustrated sheet music for Frank Wilder's

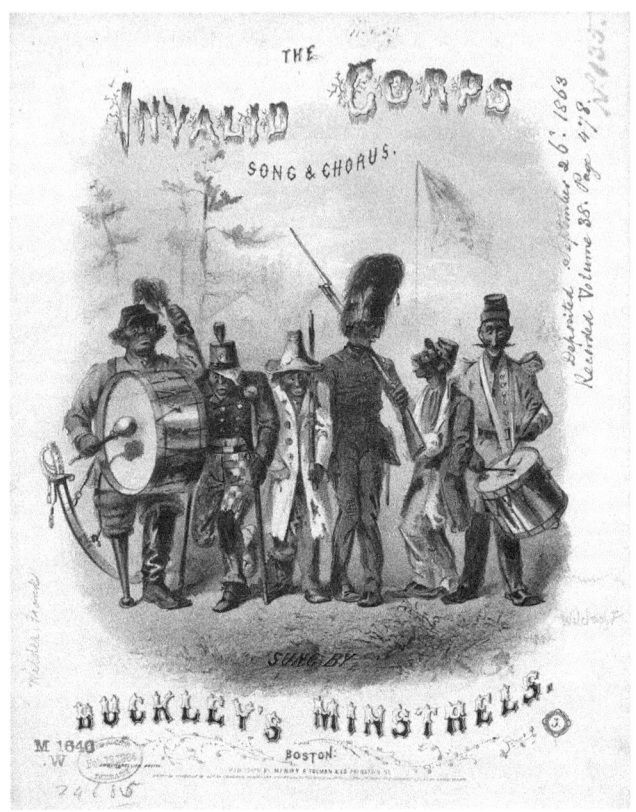

FIGURE 2. "The Invalid Corps," by Frank Wilder, published by Henry S. Tolman, Boston, 1863. Library of Congress Civil War Sheet Music Collection.

"The Invalid Corps" offers a yet deeper layer of meaning. Buckley's Minstrels, a popular blackface troupe, performed the song. The cover illustration depicts corps members as caricatures of black men.[76] These soldiers are grotesquely laughable, dressed in a mismatched assemblage of uniforms and civilian clothing. One drummer sports enormous epaulettes obviously above his rank. Another wears the trademark patchwork pants of blackface characters. In addition, the black soldiers bear various "defects," ranging from knock-knees to bandaged arms to amputated legs.

How black caricatures came to depict the Invalid Corps is a compelling question. Although the corps made some attempts to utilize disabled black soldiers, it never permitted the transfer or recruitment of black men. In the winter of 1864, Capt. Reuben Mussey, who directed the recruitment of the United States Colored Troops in the Department of the Cumberland, called for all black soldiers unfit for field duty to be placed into certain USCT regiments. Though they performed work similar to that of the white Invalid

Corps, the regiments were not designated as black companions to the corps. Nor were these units named to indicate that they were officially reserved for disabled men.[77] Later that year, Gen. Nathaniel Banks made a preliminary attempt to create a Colored Invalid Battalion, but Edwin Stanton rejected the order.[78]

Ultimately, tangled conceptions of race and disability meant that no unit officially was designated as a black Invalid Corps. White men could be disabled by degrees and still capable of some amount of work. But many believed—with the support of popular medical theories—that black men were inherently inferior and therefore rendered entirely useless by similar disabilities. Thus, the sheet music cover was not intended to depict actual black Invalid Corps soldiers. Rather, it was conceived as a manifestation of Americans' associations among manhood, blackness, and disability during the Civil War. The most visible antebellum disabilities were those of the enslaved, whose bodies bore lash marks attesting to their subjugation. During the war, the scarred black body was most famously depicted in the photograph of Gordon, an enslaved man who escaped to Union lines in the spring of 1863. Gordon's lacerated back became symbolic of slavery's brutality. Such scars were the mark of bondage, just as corporeal integrity was the mark of white male citizenship.[79]

Blackness itself was a kind of disability in antebellum America.[80] By their very nature, African Americans were judged mentally and physically inferior. In her study on black prison guards, Kelly Mezurek references records of the provost marshal general and the United States Sanitary Commission revealing that surgeons examining USCT soldiers believed them to have both "brute physical manhood" and worse health than their white counterparts.[81] The aforementioned song about the Invalid Corps appeared the same year as the USCT's establishment. At that moment, black men's ability to be soldiers was very much up for public debate. The sheet music's illustration conflates these two new portions of the Union army, suggesting that black men and disabled men make for worthless, even laughable, soldiers.

This critique cut deeper than a humorous jab. Invalid Corps members performed work that was degraded by white male standards, and they often filled the same roles as black soldiers, free blacks, or contraband. Disabled white soldiers performed hospital work alongside black men and women. Perhaps most revealing was the use of black soldiers and disabled white soldiers as prison guards at Northern prisoner of war camps. Black regiments chosen to be prison guards had proven themselves trustworthy and honorable in battle. In contrast, the white guards they served alongside

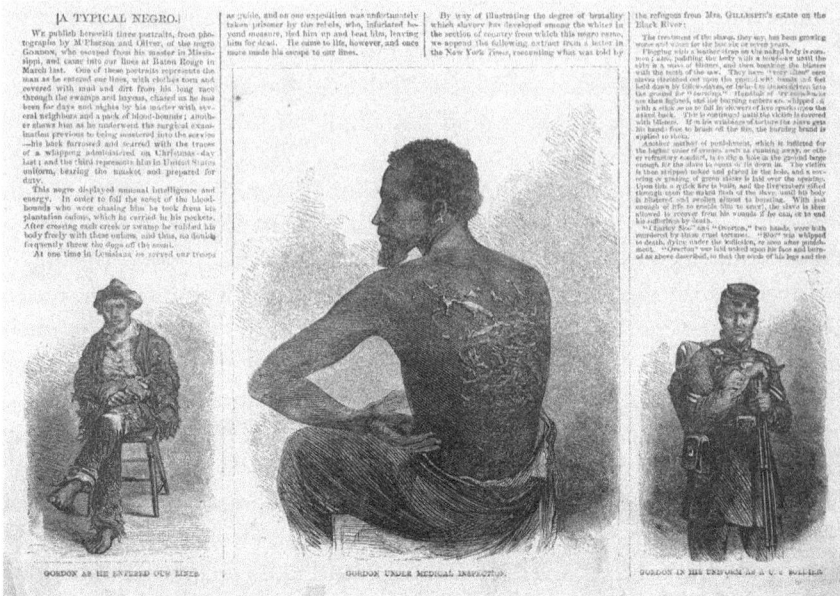

FIGURE 3. *Gordon under Medical Inspection.* Gordon's heavily scarred back is juxtaposed with images of him wearing the ragged clothes of a slave and a blue Union uniform. *Harper's Weekly,* July 4, 1863. Library of Congress.

held their positions because they were unfit. This uncomfortable juxtaposition reinforced the notion that disability placed white men in the inferior position of black men.[82] The Invalid Corps might have been created with the intention of shoring up disabled soldiers' masculinity, but in practice, it rendered it all the more vulnerable.

The Invalid Corps, both praised and mocked, captured what it meant to be a disabled white soldier in the Union army. While the corps helped to strengthen the Federal army and incapacitated soldiers filled critical support jobs, the unit's creation and implementation also revealed the contradictory reality of wartime disability. Rhetoric that fashioned war wounds into patriotic sacrifices and wounded men into heroes failed to exorcise the anxiety over disabled soldiers' manhood. Men chafed at being removed from their regiments, wearing highly identifiable new uniforms, and doing the work of women and blacks. Concern that infirmities, however honorable, could potentially make men into degraded dependents encouraged a definition of disability that tied bodies to their capacity for productive labor. As a result, disabled soldiers were forced into an awkward position between combatant and invalid.

The soldiers of the Invalid Corps might often have resented and resisted the label, but they at least benefited from one thing: a clear categorization as disabled. The corps only took men who were sick or injured badly enough to be declared unfit for field duty. However, on any given day, the ranks of the Union army were filled with footsore, coughing soldiers with aching bowels who were nonetheless judged healthy enough to serve. When they pushed too hard for accommodations, or when they made accommodations for themselves, these men—the walking sick, we might call them—came into conflict with officers, surgeons, and the military justice system.

CHAPTER 2

Army of the Walking Sick

On July 19, 1862, Pvt. Ephraim Pelton was having a bad day. He was sick and exhausted, but his commanding officers had disregarded his repeated requests for a disability discharge. Pelton found himself on guard duty for the second time in two days, standing for hours at a time and keeping watch on behalf of the rest of the unit. At some point in his shift, he closed his eyes and drifted off to sleep. This slip put him in violation of the Forty-Sixth Article of War and earned him a court-martial.[1]

Pelton was charged with sleeping at his post and brought before the court-martial board on July 25, 1862. He pleaded guilty—after all, he'd been caught sleeping and couldn't very well argue that he hadn't been—but tried to explain that it wasn't his fault. He was sick and waiting for a disability discharge. On this particular day, Pelton argued, he had been exhausted from constant guard duty and disrupted sleep. His captain and surgeon both testified on his behalf, but they didn't paint quite the picture he had hoped for. Each agreed that Pelton had indeed been sick, but the men considered it more important that he was a terrible soldier and pathetic man. Capt. O. A. Payne testified that he had never signed the paperwork for the disability discharge Pelton had requested. "He complained of rheumatism," Payne testified, "and I told him that if he would get the Doctor to write out his certificate stating his worthlessness and inability on account of manhood to make a good soldier, I would give him his discharge." Unsurprisingly, Pelton was found guilty and sentenced to thirty days' hard labor and the loss of one month's pay. It is telling that Pelton's punishment was more work, as if manual labor could rehabilitate his weakness and inferior manhood.[2]

Many Union soldiers found themselves in Pelton's quandary at some point during their service: neither sick enough to warrant a hospital stay or discharge nor well enough to meet the expectations of able-bodiedness military service demanded. Relief was available for overtly ill soldiers, who could report sick and get extra rest or a trip to the hospital to recuperate. Those suffering from imprecise or common ailments were often deemed lazy or, worse, accused of malingering. Unlike the disabled men who believed their segregation into the Invalid Corps was unjust, the walking sick strove to inform officers that they were *more* impaired rather than less.

Military manhood depended on adherence to the demands of wartime's unique expectations—respecting authority, following orders, completing duties without complaint. None of these requirements had to be fulfilled in such exacting terms in soldiers' civilian lives. Pain and sickness made meeting these expectations more difficult.[3] Soldiers who insisted on accommodations for their ailing bodies, or who were unable to overcome their physical infirmities and continue serving, risked being accused of lacking masculine resolve. The result was a difficult situation for disabled soldiers. In order to continue serving in their units, men bent to the needs of their bodies by straggling, leaving their posts, or otherwise violating the Articles of War. When they did so, they came into conflict with officers, surgeons, and court-martial boards. These interactions revealed another layer of the contest over who had the authority to define what it meant to be able and unable. Soldiers asserted the evidence of their own bodies; officers and surgeons asserted their rank. While officers sometimes agreed with ailing soldiers, it was officers' authority that ultimately determined what counted as a disability.

The experiences of the walking sick also broaden our understanding of wartime disability. Civil War disability is most closely associated with battle wounds, particularly amputation, but disability from illness was a far more common experience. Though modern scholars often distinguish between ill health and impairment, Union army officials understood illness as a form of disability. Discharge papers for incapacitated soldiers drew no distinctions between disease and injuries. Far more disability discharges were granted for disease than for war wounds. For those who remained in the army, the Invalid Corps made the overlap between illness and disability apparent. As noted in the previous chapter, the majority of enlisted corps members were declared unfit for field service and disabled due to disease or chronic illness.[4] While there are legitimate reasons to interpret illness and disability differently, the soldiers, officers, and surgeons of the Union army considered them critically interrelated. Such was the case even when illness caused temporary impairment.[5] Sick soldiers, just like those incapacitated by war wounds, were sometimes unable to meet the expectations of military service. In many cases, they sought disability status so they could access care or rest. The trials of the walking sick offer evidence for a redefinition of Civil War disability and a reassessment of the war's impact on the bodies of its combatants.

Ephraim Pelton's trial centered on the question of whether he had truly been too ill to keep awake, or whether he was a bad soldier and weak man. Unbeknownst to the ailing Pelton, his case was part of a larger dialogue within the Union army over bodies, health, and military discipline. When soldiers used their bodies as an explanation for their crimes, they came up against commanders concerned about poor discipline, increasing absenteeism, and dwindling morale. These superior officers adjudicated not only the soldier's guilt or innocence but also the legitimacy of their disability and the potency of their manhood.

Scholars of desertion and straggling identify a number of reasons why soldiers chose to leave the ranks, whether temporarily or permanently. Though many have discussed the role that physical discomfort played in desertions, few have specifically explored the relationship between health and absenteeism.[6] Kathryn Shively's recent study considers the ways that average soldiers used straggling—temporarily leaving the ranks with the intention of returning—as a form of self-care during the 1862 Peninsula Campaign.[7] Shively concludes that straggling was often a response to soldiers' bodily needs, rather than a reflection of poor discipline, low morale, or cowardice. In order to continue in service, soldiers sometimes felt they needed to leave camp for a night in a dry barn, a hot meal, or nursing from a woman in a nearby village.[8] These men considered straggling a necessary part of successful soldiering, and they did not associate it with cowardice or lack of discipline. Officers, on the other hand, often distrusted soldiers' claims of pain or ill health, believing such behavior indicated inferior martial masculinity.

Not all officers equated shirking or straggling with cowardice. Lower-ranking and noncommissioned officers were more sympathetic to the common soldiers' complaints, but high-ranking officers, concerned about waning manpower, believed stragglers were proving their weak character by failing to "man up" and do their duty. Cultural and class differences, as well as conflicting ideas about military bearing, often accounted for differing ideas about military manhood. Most in the upper echelons of the officer ranks had come from the regular army. They therefore held strict beliefs about soldierly behavior and doubted volunteers' ability to endure the difficulties of military life.[9] The disagreement over how to deal with absenteeism led to a crackdown on straggling and absenteeism in the Confederate and Federal armies in 1862. Commanders required lower-ranking officers and surgeons to carefully scrutinize the sick and provide sick leave or furloughs only when absolutely necessary. Increasingly strict punishments were recommended for those caught out of ranks.[10]

As the creation of the Invalid Corps indicated, many in the Union army believed that disability discharges were given too generously early in the war, and that soldiers abused the system. Complaining that only a fraction of furloughed soldiers ever returned, commanders believed some men used an illness or wound as an excuse to go to the hospital, only to sneak away home.[11] Of course, some soldiers did try to game the system. Christian Lenker, sergeant in the Nineteenth Ohio, recalled soldiers flocking to the doctor each evening when he inspected men for furloughs after the Battle of Shiloh. "Many of the men should have been to the 'front' but some were homesick and 'played off' trying to get a discharge or furlough."[12] Even Abraham Lincoln expressed concern at the high rate of disabled absentees in Gen. George McClellan's Army of the Potomac during the 1862 Peninsula Campaign. The president suggested that most of these soldiers were likely "fit for duty."[13] Whether or not this impression was entirely accurate, a level of distrust surrounded soldiers who sought leave or disability discharges.

The perception that soldiers were taking advantage of furloughs prompted the War Department to issue new leave policies in June 1862. Together, the orders made it difficult to obtain a furlough and to use health as an excuse for a late return. General Order 61 disallowed anyone but the secretary of war, or in dire cases the commander of an army, department, or district, from authorizing leave. General Order 65 designated that all men away from their units be declared deserters, with no leniency extended for stragglers or those who overstayed a furlough. The order also made it clear that illness was not an acceptable excuse for absence.[14]

This strict policy only lasted a few months. In January 1863, as part of a campaign to improve morale in the Army of the Potomac, Maj. Gen. Joe Hooker relaxed the furlough policy. Leaves were granted to men with excellent records, and soldiers could only leave when the previous man returned. If even one soldier overstayed his leave, the entire company could lose the right to furloughs—a powerful deterrent.[15] The change improved troops' spirits, and many soldiers took it seriously. However, these modifications did not change the policy of treating late returners claiming sickness as deserters. Hooker's requirements made furloughs more accessible. Even so, leave was often promised weeks in advance, making it difficult to use the time to recover from illnesses. Sympathetic soldiers swapped their furloughs with desperate comrades in some cases, but it generally remained difficult to get leave for ailments that weren't severe. As one New Jersey soldier wrote his sister in 1863, "I might as well try to fly as to try to get a furlough."[16]

Tighter control over what ailments merited a discharge and suspicion that soldiers gamed the system for light duty or time off meant that many surgeons only offered extra rest to those with severe ailments. But almost all soldiers became sick at some point during their service, though not all them would require hospitalization. For these walking sick, the needs of the human body and the requirements of the Union army were often at odds. Thus soldiers found themselves in the difficult position of trying to prove they were as sick as they claimed. Transcripts from courts-martial in which health was under debate offer a glimpse into this army of the walking sick, and into the negotiations between soldiers and the authorities. The small sample of courts-martial presented in this chapter spanned the war years and took place in both the Eastern and Western Theaters. Each source makes reference to the health of the soldier—sometimes in his own words, sometimes in the testimony of witnesses. The men in these cases were charged with various infractions, ranging from the relatively minor (such as sleeping on post) to the very serious (desertion).

At the center of these courts-martial lay the conflict between soldiers' perceptions of their own bodies and authorities' conclusions about their bodies. While soldiers believed their embodied experience should suffice as an alibi, officers and surgeons countered with the expectations of military manhood. The outcomes of these trials were mixed. When officers sympathized with the soldier's story and felt assured of his good character, they were ready to offer lighter punishment or, on occasion, dismiss charges. Less scrupulous soldiers aware of this situation doubtless attempted exaggerating symptoms to gain favor. But evidence suggests that in more cases, ailing soldiers genuinely struggled to keep up or stay at it. Officers were not always quite so understanding. When they took offense at perceived evidence of cowardice, insufficient manhood, or malingering, officers meted out harsh or humiliating punishments. Whether a man was found guilty or innocent, the arguments raised in courts-martial revealed soldiers' and officers' differing, often conflicting definitions of disability, as well as the cultural assumptions about manhood and ability that informed those debates.

Sick soldiers charged with desertion or being absent without leave protested that they needed care or rest. Even when they knew that leaving violated military order, it still seemed sensible to seek a respite. Volunteer soldiers continued to think like civilians, and in their premilitary experience, sickness had meant avoiding exposure to severe weather, finding nourishing food, and getting rest. Steven Ramold describes the conflict that often arose between citizen-soldiers and the regular army over straightforward matters in the civilian world, such as speaking frankly or resisting poor leaders' authority.[17] Ill health constituted another instance where soldiers acted in ways that made sense in their civilian lives but violated codes of military order.

Though soldiers often admitted awareness of breaking the rules, they believed that their bodies would exonerate them. Pvt. David Okes, for example, was charged with desertion in September 1862 after he left camp with an ill-gotten pass and failed to return for thirty days. He had not attempted to shirk duty until suffering a "sprained or dislocated ankle" in June 1862.[18] Witnesses explained that Okes had tried and failed to get a furlough from the regimental surgeon on account of his "sore feet." Then he had made his mind up to leave anyway. Okes eventually found an army provost he could pay off in exchange for a pass, which he used to travel home for some rest. After thirty days, presumably when his ankle was feeling better, he returned to his regiment, ready to resume his duties.[19] Okes understood that he had violated the Articles of War. Yet he also seemed to believe that taking a respite was the only way he could continue to serve.

Other soldiers only fell out for short periods of rest. Pvt. Alexander Cranston, feeling unwell, left the front lines to escape the rain for a few hours and warm himself by the fire. He fully intended to rejoin the regiment in the morning, but a provost guard arrested him.[20] In another instance, Pvt. Thomas F. Fenlan found himself unable to keep up on the march after four days on the sick list. He fell out and "left the Regt to go to a house to get warm." A few days later, he tried to rejoin the regiment but could not find his superior officer. Fenlan then decided to find a warm meal while he waited for the lieutenant to return to his tent. In his search for some hoecake, Fenlan was discovered and arrested as a deserter.[21]

Even when they were obviously culpable, soldiers sometimes tried to pin their actions on the authorities who refused to accommodate them. Dennis Kelley tried to get on the sick list through the regimental surgeon's recommendation several times, but each time was found fit for duty. Kelley explained to the court that he had been suffering from chronic bleeding—though from where and why somehow went unrecorded. In the winter of 1863, after a sleepless, bloody night, Kelley reported sick yet again. The exasperated surgeon could do nothing for him. Kelley thought he saw the surgeon write "duty" on the sick list, so when the surgeon wasn't looking, Kelley took the list, rubbed out the word, and marked himself down as sick. In his desperation, Kelley had not seen that the surgeon had actually marked him down for a day of rest in his quarters. For his moment of panic, Kelley was court-martialed. In his statement to the board, he admitted his actions but placed the real blame on the surgeon. Kelley might have been technically guilty, but the exhaustion and excitement caused by continued duty had made him insensible.[22]

For the most part, soldiers did their best to keep working, even when their bodies were at their limit. Like Ephraim Pelton, these men were charged with crimes not because they straggled or shirked, but because they had been denied care and their ailing bodies simply had not allowed them to perform their required duties. Pvt. Edward Stratton was suffering from a nasty case of seasickness while on the voyage from New York State to Baton Rouge, Louisiana. However, he was still required to keep guard for twenty-four hours, standing sentry for two hours and then taking four hours off. When the boat arrived in Baton Rouge, Stratton was immediately placed on picket duty, where he was to stand guard every two hours for two hours at a time. Sick and exhausted, he had a dizzy spell, dozed off, and was promptly charged with sleeping on his post.

Falling asleep on post and leaving a post momentarily were common charges for sick soldiers, especially those suffering from the scourge of soldierly life, diarrhea. Both Elso Boelson and Thomas Jaeger were charged with sleeping on post, and each man attributed his momentary weakness to painful bowels. Boelson knew his regiment was already suffering from low manpower and so made up his mind "to do [his] duty without complaint." He did not remember falling asleep, but he admitted the possibility because he had been "very weak and exhausted by exposure."[23] Jaegar explained that he had experienced an attack of colic that might have caused him to fall asleep on duty.[24] Poor Henry Peers found himself in an even more compromising position. Also dealing with diarrhea, Peers told his fellow picket that he was just leaving his post for a moment to relieve himself. He walked twenty yards away and returned within moments, only to find his unsympathetic captain waiting for him.[25]

Today, historical understanding of sickness in the Union army relies on *The Medical and Surgical History of the War of the Rebellion (MSHWR)*, the official records of Federal soldiers' and officers' injuries and diseases. While an irreplaceable resource, the *MSHWR* suffers from all the expected problems of Civil War record keeping: underreporting, missing records, selective notations. For the study of the soldiers serving while impaired, the work suffers from another significant flaw—it only concerns those sick enough to warrant a surgeon's care, hospitalization, or discharge. Men like Elso

Boelson, Thomas Jaeger, and Henry Peers, who considered themselves unwell but went undiagnosed, and who were not quite sick enough to warrant direct care or medical leave, are not represented.

Further, the *MSHWR* only includes those cases surgeons considered important enough to record. It's doubtful that doctors noted each soldier complaining of headache or sore feet, or each soldier suffering from the ubiquitous bowel complaint. The *MSHWR* records nearly 1.5 million cases of diarrhea, meaning that over half the Union army suffered from the ailment severely enough to merit a surgeon's report. Yet most agree that number is still low. With so many rampant diarrheal illnesses, far more soldiers presumably suffered to some extent at one point or another.[26] Anecdotal evidence seems to bear out this assertion. Bell Wiley suggests that although references to sick soldiers abound in diaries and letters, their recorded numbers might have been low because many of them chose not to report to a surgeon.[27] In Kathryn Shively's sample of the letters and diaries of troops serving in Virginia in 1862, only 15 percent of the men were consistently healthy. Thus almost all of the soldiers in the sample reported feeling sick or demoralized at least once.[28] The records show that the numbers of soldiers who died or suffered from disease during the Civil War are staggering, so it seems likely that the numbers of men who felt unwell at one point or another must be truly huge.

It seems reasonable to conclude, then, that almost all soldiers felt sick at some point, but that most were not hospitalized or placed on the sick list. Instead, they continued to perform field duty while ailing. Despite the ubiquity of sickness, soldiers who complained too loudly of their bodily ills were often suspected of malingering—manufacturing or faking an ailment with the aim of getting out of duty—or accused of lacking proper masculine military resolve. After all, the military and civilian population alike reserved the highest praise for soldiers who suffered manfully through wounds and pain. Frances Clarke describes the proliferation of popular media stories about soldiers bearing their suffering with fortitude. Americans came to expect soldiers to have "pluck," a characteristic that allowed soldiers to bear pain or suffering with something like cheer, even in dire circumstances. As an example, Clarke points to Gen. Dan Sickles, who apparently gave a witty speech to his men after losing his leg at the Battle of Gettysburg. While addressing the troops, he referred to his catastrophic injury as a "little inconvenience."[29]

Sickles stands out, of course, because of his generalship, but the same kind of courage came to be expected of all sick and wounded men. Ideal citizen-soldiers manfully suffered in the name of their country. So when soldiers seeking relief requested a discharge or light duty, they admitted to feeling less than cheery about their bodily privations, violating expectations of martial masculinity. Soldiering with an impairment meant walking the fine line between manhood and disgrace. As one Michigan soldier warned, a man who could not handle the hardships of war "had better pack his knapsack and gow home to his mother."[30] But soldiers and officers often had competing ideas about what it meant to properly withstand the hardships of war. Soldiers did not believe that seeking comfort was incompatible with the standards of manhood. Rather, they believed they needed to be healthy to serve well. Officers often escaped the physical privations that plagued enlisted men; for instance, they had warmer, dryer quarters or a horse to ride while on the march. Therefore, officers were more likely to interpret troops' inability to withstand hardships as evidence of poor character and clear violations of military law.[31]

Men who lacked pluck risked accusations of malingering. Few soldiers were officially charged with malingering in courts-martial, but explicit and implicit allegations often emerged in court testimony. Whether or not a soldier was truly ill, his attempts to get medical care could suggest poor character and be interpreted as evidence of malingering. The *MSHWR* recorded surgeons' burden of identifying fakers, relating that there was "scarcely a regimental medical officer whose experience did not include the persistent efforts of one or more men to be relieved from the dangers of field service by transfer to general hospital or discharge on certificate of disability."[32]

The court-martial of James McGrogan, member of the Sixty-Second New York, demonstrates the risks of complaining too much. McGrogan had gone missing from his unit on the hard march to Gettysburg on June 29. He claimed that he had been ill but that the march had made it impossible to get a pass from a surgeon. He had taken it upon himself to gain admittance to a hospital, remaining there until provost marshal guards discovered him. Although McGrogan had been in the hospital for some time, the guards distrusted his claims of rheumatism and ague. Two officers from the Sixty-Second testified to McGrogan's reputation for complaining and straggling. McGrogan's sergeant testified that he was "always complaining of being sick," and his captain stated that he had routinely struggled to keep up on marches.[33] While they didn't specifically accuse him of malingering, their language made the charge fairly clear.

Malingering was a real phenomenon that tempted soldiers and troubled physicians. Soldiers turned to feigning ill health for a number of reasons, including concerns about loved ones at home. Doubting her fidelity, one soldier wrote to his wife of the lengths he was taking to get out of the service: "I want to get out of this thing some way if I can. . . . When you write I wish you would send me some Arsnic or some other kind of stuff so as to make me look pale . . . find out at the druggist what will make you look pale and sickly."[34] James McGrogan's case contained the implied allegation that he chose to leave on the night of June 30, 1863, because he knew a big fight was coming. It was commonly agreed that soldiers often suddenly developed an infirmity on the eve of a battle.[35] Scared, tired, and sick, they shot off fingers and toes, swallowed poisons, feigned a bad back—anything that might earn them a ticket home.[36] The statistical prevalence of malingering is nearly impossible to determine. But anecdotal evidence offers numerous stories of soldiers who were caught out by clever, and maybe a touch sadistic, surgeons threatening to drown, burn, and otherwise torture suspected malingerers into recanting.[37]

These dramatic stories present physicians as patriotic professionals doggedly rooting out craven and malicious pretenders. Certainly, outing fakers helped to strengthen the fighting force and protect morale. At the same time, it's critical to remember the source of most of these anecdotes—officers and surgeons who were on the lookout for troublesome soldiers, and who distrusted those whose demands for medical attention were too loud or persistent. It's more than possible that some reports were cases of hammer-wielding physicians seeing so many nails. Some legitimate ailments could easily have been interpreted as malingering—rheumatism, for example, one of James McGrogan's ailments, was a common target. The *MSHWR* noted that chronic rheumatism seemed particularly appealing to malingerers because of its "subjective symptoms."[38] Claiming rheumatism became so notorious by the summer of 1862 that it was the only ailment General Order 65 specifically designated off-limits for disability discharge.[39] William Fuller, surgeon of the First Michigan Infantry, singled out rheumatism in a medical school thesis, warning surgeons trying to out its sufferers, "You may blister, cup . . . and burn them, [but] they will still persist in their assertions."[40]

While malicious soldiers could certainly have used the catchall ailment, it's also possible that combatants self-diagnosed their real but hard-to-define physical discomforts as rheumatism. The aches and pains that came with sleeping rough, marching long distances, and lacking adequate food and shelter fit into soldiers' conception of the ailment.[41] Whether surgeons deemed their symptoms a true case of rheumatism did not lessen soldiers' experience of those symptoms. Rheumatism was difficult to diagnose. It left few physical signs on the body, and surgeons had to rely largely on soldiers' testimony to identify it. In addition, while a soldier had to rely on words to get a surgeon to believe him, most surgeons interpreted such self-advocacy as evidence of weak manhood and an attempt to get out of service. Roberts Bartholow admitted that pain was not visible. Even so, he insisted that real rheumatics would offer some visual proof of the disease through swelling, wasting, or overall poor appearance. "When the health is good and the seat of the alleged pain is unaffected by swelling or increased temperature," Bartholow quoted from another text, "a medical officer will probably in nineteen out of twenty cases be safe in concluding that no material, or at any rate, no permanent disease exists."[42] Rheumatism drew the most ire, but all nonvisible impairments, such as back pain, headache, and lung disease, were linked to malingering.

Heart disease was also considered a common ailment used by malingerers. Bartholow remained convinced that almost all heart-related complaints were faked, except in very particular cases. Most heart disease, he maintained, came from poor character: "Functional derangement of the heart is produced by various evil habits—excessive tobacco-chewing, indigestion, masturbation, much of the time being passed in bed . . . and finally, nostalgia."[43] Heart palpitations could be feigned just by feeling emotions too fervently. Bartholow's description insinuates that men complaining of heart ailments were cowardly, immoral, and feminine. Jacob DaCosta, an expert on heart disease who identified irritable heart, the ailment unique to overburdened soldiers, dismissed accusations that heart disease was easily feigned. He instead suggested that appropriate testing by a trained physician could differentiate an exaggerated case from a true one.[44]

Surgeons were counseled to be vigilant about identifying potential fakers. Bartholow suggested, "As a rule, it is better for the military surgeon, in all cases of doubt, to suspect any soldier of feigning whose symptoms are obscure, unreasonable, or improbable." However, a surgeon should also play along with such patients until his suspicions were confirmed. While physicians often attempted to reveal fakers by using painful or unpleasant "treatments," this plan did not always work as intended. One private from an Illinois regiment "complained of his back, breast, and legs; in fact, every part of him has at one time or another been the seat of trouble," his frustrated surgeon stated. Even after being treated with "cups, blisters, tonics, strychnia, and colchieum, full diet and plenty of exercise," the man's condition failed to improve.[45] The surgeon quipped cynically, "He is one of a kind that cannot be cured while in the military service."[46] That the ailment was real and his cures were worthless, the surgeon did not consider.

Despite insistence from medical authorities like Bartholow that malingerers were rampant, not all surgeons were quick to assume soldiers were faking. When describing "pernicious fever," surgeon G. Rush noted that unusual, fast-developing symptoms sometimes meant that doctors accused sufferers of malingering before realizing they were seriously ill.[47] Another surgeon suggested that medical officers who were not practiced enough in diagnosing illnesses were too quick to condemn a soldier as a malingerer. "It is very common for medical officers, when they do not understand the disease, to accuse the soldier of *malingering*, in regard to night-blindness, many considered all cases feigned," reported surgeon J. C. Norton in 1861. He continued, "I am aware that when a disease becomes popular there are many soldiers who will take advantage of it and feign the symptoms to avoid duty. At the same time, my observation has taught me that there is not one-half as much malingering in the army as is generally supposed."[48]

Who was correct in his assessment of malingering within the Union army: Bartholow, who believed malingerers lurked in every corner, or Norton, who suspected reports were overblown? The answer depends on who we believe had the power to legitimize disability. In James McGrogan's case, his superior officers attempted to discredit his ailments, while the soldier himself maintained the validity of his suffering. And though it wasn't always the situation, in this case, the court-martial board awarded McGrogan the ultimate authority. He was found not guilty of desertion, and he returned to service in his unit.[49]

A month after the Battle of Antietam, while the Nineteenth United States was still encamped near the battlefield, Pvt. Peter Boyer left the regiment and trekked home to Somerset County, Pennsylvania. When he was arrested a few weeks later in his mother's home, he stated simply that he had left the ranks because he had been homesick. When the arresting officer warned him that he would be "punished severely for what he had done," Boyer said he didn't care and would "stand the punishment." The desire to be at home, even for a short time, was worth the penalty.[50]

While Peter Boyer didn't have a label for his intense homesickness, thousands of soldiers did. The medical diagnosis of nostalgia paired debilitating homesickness with symptoms similar to modern-day depression.[51] Although Civil War–era physicians believed nostalgia was a genuine illness, many also believed it plagued men incapable of adhering to the expectations of military manhood.[52] Surgeon John L. Taylor of the Third Missouri Cavalry took this point particularly seriously. Nostalgic patients, he believed, were pathologically weak, immoral, and cowardly: "The home-sick patient shows a want of resolution and activity in all his undertakings; he is serious, sad, and timid, apprehending on the slightest grounds the most serious results—great personal danger, and even death itself. This condition is soon followed by emaciation, languor and listlessness." Taylor held that patients brought these symptoms on themselves.

The belief persisted that nostalgia manifested itself only in men who were already weak willed, men whose lack of manly resolve allowed the disease to ravage their bodies and minds. As Frances Clarke argues, willpower was a critical component of manhood. Failing to control one's homesick feelings, then, was the mark of a poor man.[53] Moreover, this weakness was, in a sense, contagious. If surgeons allowed nostalgic patients to be discharged for the illness, Taylor wrote, it would "encourage others to indulge in the hope of getting away."[54] Merely contemplating others' nostalgia could cause a case of nostalgia, which, in turn, indicated a soldier's moral inferiority and weakness.

Nostalgia and malingering were tightly intertwined.[55] Nostalgic soldiers stubbornly insisted that they were sick, and believed that their illness warranted a trip home. Doctors asserted that men with nostalgia suffered from "hypochondriasis," a male hysteria resulting in imprecise symptoms such as "palpitations," "morbid feelings," and "panics." Here again, soldiers and physicians disagreed over who had the proper authority to decide one's illness or health. Many soldiers, Taylor grumbled, "exaggerated uneasiness of various kinds, chiefly in regards [to their] health, which they strenuously contended was seriously injured and could not be restored short of being at home."[56] Soldiers who stuck to their guns over their "strenuous contentions" frustrated physicians who thought self-diagnoses undermined professional authority.

Nostalgic men, like malingerers, were criticized for failing to bear illness with the appropriate masculine "pluck." Taylor believed that nostalgic patients were not inclined to be active in curing their illness. Instead, "there was a stubborn indolence in these patients," who were "generally found lying in bed or sitting around the tents, making a great deal to do about their sufferings and the ills that were awaiting them." Like malingerers, nostalgia sufferers insisted too fervently on their sickness. In order to force soldiers out of their doldrums, Taylor prescribed daily physical exercise and instituted a campaign to shame them into health. He initiated a policy to "impress [nostalgic soldiers] that their disease was a moral turpitude; that soldiers of courage, patriotism, and sense should be superior to the influences that [had] brought about their condition, and that to speak of home as inseparably connected with their recovery, and all that constituted happiness, was petty and degenerating."

Taylor even went so far as to train his nurses to treat cases of nostalgia with utter contempt. They were to act with the understanding "that gonorrhea and syphilis were not more detestable." It was not the illness that disgusted Taylor, but the weakness and degraded manhood. Nostalgic soldiers' utter lack of pluck proved that they were pathetic and unable (or unwilling) to overcome what was considered an indulgent illness. Surely such men could not be true Union soldiers "superior to the influences that [had] brought about their condition."[57] A combatant's ability to bear up to the trials of warfare telegraphed important messages about his character, and a man who complained, asked for accommodation, or broke down was no man at all.

When a soldier's health brought him not to the hospital but before the court-martial board, the question of what counted as a legitimate disability—and who made that decision—became a matter of great importance. As demonstrated by the wartime conversations about malingering and nostalgia, soldiers often believed their suffering was enough to warrant light duty or time off. Skeptical officers and surgeons then countered with accusations of exaggerating, faking, or being too weak to bear up to the expectations of soldiering. The more insistently soldiers voiced their need for rest, warmth, food, or furloughs, the more convinced their officers became of their unworthiness. At the core of this tension was a disagreement over what constituted a disability.

Court-martial boards required evidence, but what evidence held weight? Soldiers believed in the facts of their own experience, but officers and surgeons believed in what could be seen or clearly diagnosed—in other words, were there obvious wounds or overt signs of sickness? Evidence of the soldier's character was just as important. Court-martial boards, like commanding officers and surgeons, were more likely to give the benefit of the doubt to a soldier who performed his duty well. Ephraim Pelton's dilemma is illustrative. He felt sick, but his superiors believed he appeared healthy enough to keep serving. Instead of pushing through his discomfort, Pelton asked for a discharge, which communicated to his officers that he was a poor soldier. Perhaps Pelton was. But the claim of impairment was at issue, and it was a matter of his word against his superiors'.

The case of John O'Niel, a member of the First New York Volunteer Engineers, offers a powerful example of how a question of health could spark conflict between enlisted men and officers. When Capt. F. E. Graaf tried to get an unruly O'Niel to quiet down and go to bed after tattoo in April 1862, O'Niel responded with a string of obscenities. The soldier had a reputation for being stubborn and sometimes difficult, and he was no great fan of his commanding officer. When Graaf insisted again that O'Niel be quiet, O'Niel tried to punch the captain in the face and clipped him in the chin. Convinced that the man was drunk, Graaf and his fellow officers had him arrested. O'Niel's tent mates testified that he had not been drinking. Rather, he had been loud and irritable because he was nearly mad with the intense pain of "the gravel" (kidney stones). A surgical procedure a few days later to remove the stone proved this claim. Nevertheless, O'Niel was found guilty, partly because of the severity of his outburst, and partly because of his bad reputation.[58] The case demonstrates the strength of the word of an officer versus that of a troublesome enlisted man. Though O'Niel and several comrades testified to his intense pain, and his condition was borne out by surgery, Captain Graaf's erroneous allegation of drunkenness (and no doubt his anger at being struck and insulted by a private) carried more weight.

Unfortunately for Private O'Niel, no matter how painful his kidney stone was, it was invisible to his superior officers. Even when a surgeon confirmed O'Neil's claims, his loud and unruly conduct while suffering proved his poor bearing as a soldier. Court-martial boards, however, occasionally extended sympathy to a man who exhibited such behavior. When Pvt. Michael Young of the Second Battalion of the Invalid Corps was court-martialed in 1863, he faced some serious charges: drunkenness, disobeying orders, and conduct prejudicial to good order and military discipline. The soldier had been in trouble for leaving his post before and was known for being surly. In late October 1863, Young was seen drinking heavily in a nearby town. Later, he was observed resting on a bench while on duty. When his captain ordered him to the guardhouse, Young lashed out with strong language and his cane, striking at the unfortunate sergeant trying to arrest him.

Even witnesses called in Young's defense could only do so much. When asked about Young's soldierly qualities, Sgt. Albert Zandtler testified bluntly, "He is a good man when he is not drunk." It seemed a pretty cut-and-dried case; Young pled guilty to all charges except that of conduct prejudicial, and the court obligingly found him guilty on all counts. Yet the private was only required to forfeit a few months' pay. "The court [is] thus lenient," its members explained, "because of the crippled condition of the prisoner, he having lost his right leg in the service—amputated above the knee." Unlike O'Niel, Young had a highly visible disability and proof of a previous sacrifice, which the officers of the court-martial board deemed an acceptable excuse for his behavior. In this case, it was not the soldier or officer who offered the most powerful testimony—it was the obvious and incontrovertible absence of a limb.

For surgeons and officers, moments like these—when a soldier faced pain, discomfort, or anguish—held the potential to separate true soldiers from emasculated and immoral ones. Those who could not meet the expectations of martial manhood in the difficult moments demonstrated themselves to be, in the language of both fellow soldiers and the civilian public, cowards, malingerers, and mercenaries. In short, these men were the opposite of true-blue Union volunteers. Roberts Bartholow believed that few malingerers came from the ranks of genuine (read white middle-class) volunteers, but instead were Irish, German, or working-class Americans who "were induced to enter service . . . by a sudden zeal which had no foundation in a conviction of duty, or by the stimulus of a large bounty."[59] True soldiers of the Union selflessly gave themselves to the jaws of war purely out of devotion to the cause. They handled moments of suffering with masculine composure and cheerful resolve.

Stories of idealized Union soldiers who bore suffering with grace became commonplace in the civilian media. War correspondents and editorialists praised the Union combatant for bearing pain with a smile. One journalist reporting on wounded soldiers on a hospital ship described a young man with "three balls in each leg, both arms broken, and back badly bruised" who was nevertheless in "good spirits," even joking with his nurses.[60] How soldiers coped with an injury or sickness revealed a great deal. "By commendably bearing their illnesses and injuries," writes Frances Clarke, "they revealed the strength of their characters, the force of their religion, and the depths of their civic commitment."[61] But not all soldiers could meet this expectation. With the belief that all *true* soldiers experienced pain and suffering with the bravery displayed by the wounded soldier on that hospital steamer, those who whined or sought a discharge or admitted the negative effects of an impairment could never fit into that category. Thus, when the suffering Ephraim Pelton asked for a disability discharge, his superior officer offered him one—but only if he signed a document declaring him unfit for duty due to inferior manhood.

In recent years, historians have begun pushing Civil War medical history beyond the testimony of physicians and authority figures to include the perspectives of patients.[62] In order to create a truly popular medical history of the Civil War, we have to grapple with the power dynamics at play as officers, surgeons, and soldiers attempted to define health and impairment. While historians have long recognized the toll soldiering took on the body, we have sometimes privileged the testimony of the surgeons and officers over the words of soldiers who seemed to be shirking their duties. Undoubtedly, some soldiers exaggerated symptoms, feigned ailments, or had legitimately poor service records. But to dismiss the testimony of soldiers, even those with poor records, offering the evidence of their own bodies threatens to reproduce this power differential within the pages of our histories. Indeed, lending credence to disabled people's words is a bedrock principle of disability history.

Recorded in court-martial documents, the words of the walking sick reveal a fighting force not only sicker than previously assessed, but also divided over what kinds of ailments counted as disabilities, and who had the power to make that determination. Soldiers whose conditions did not warrant hospitalization or sick leave struggled to meet the physical demands of the army. When they were unable to do so, or when they practiced self-care by straggling, men often found themselves facing court-martial. Soldiers who advocated too loudly for their health were ostracized as weak willed, immoral, and unmanly.

The distinction between good and bad soldiers had far-reaching consequences. In a practical sense, soldiers who ran afoul of military justice struggled to get any pension benefits following the war. But in broader terms, many in and out of the army emerged from the war believing that the soldiers who had really saved the Union fit idealized standards of military manhood. Malingerers, the weak willed, and those who lacked character were merely hangers-on. As soldiers became veterans and sought pensions for their war-related ailments, they were again sorted into these categories. Like those who complained or requested extra rest, veterans who advocated too stridently for their pensions were quickly explained away as bad soldiers. Authority figures and average soldiers once again found themselves conflicted over what constituted a true war-related disability. The two groups had vastly different standards for evidence. Just as court-martial boards adjudged John O'Niel's kidney stone and Michael Young's amputated leg very differently, pension bureaucrats categorized soldiers based on their personal beliefs about the validity of the men's claims of disability, and their opinions of the men's reputation and character.

Determining who had the ultimate authority over disabled bodies could also have more immediate—and more intimate—consequences. While soldiers who straggled or failed to do their duty found themselves in conflict with military justice, some sick and wounded soldiers found themselves in conflict with the very men tasked with curing them. Dead soldiers had no power at all, leaving their corpses behind for medical professionals to use as they would. As Union doctors began to think about the medical legacies the war would leave, another question arose: Who had authority over the bodies—and body parts—of disabled soldiers?

CHAPTER 3

The United States Government Is Entitled to All of You

Sometime in 1863 or 1864, a young Union soldier visited the newly established Army Medical Museum in Washington, DC. The museum was to be a repository for the medical history of the Civil War, filled with bones, preserved lengths of bowel, sketches of dying men, and the like. The soldier politely requested help finding his amputated limb, which was on display. Dr. John Brinton, curator of the museum, later recalled that an assistant curator found the limb easily and allowed the man to view it. But the soldier was not content to simply visit his limb—he wanted it back. It belonged to him, or so he believed. "It seemed to him," wrote Brinton, "his own property and he demanded it noisily and pertinaciously. He was deaf to reason." Unmoved by the soldier's desire to reclaim his lost property, the assistant began to question him: "'For how long did you enlist, for three years or for the war?' The answer was 'For the war.' 'The United States Government is entitled to all of you, until the expiration of the specified time. I dare not give a part of you up before. Come, *then*, and you can have the rest of you, but not before.' He [the soldier] went away silently, wiser, but not convinced."[1] "So you see," Brinton observed, "that even dry bones may be regarded from different points of view."[2]

Previous chapters outline how disabled soldiers' bodies were a site of contention over the parameters of white manhood and the definitions of impairment. In the case of members of the Invalid Corps and the walking sick, soldiers remained useful as long as they could serve a purpose in the ranks. Yet incapacitated men—even dead ones—could also continue to be of use. As many historians demonstrate, the bodies of living and dead Union soldiers were critical to crafting the collective memory of the war. In political rhetoric and popular media, and as part of the creation of commemorative spaces and occasions, soldiers' bodies served as tools for understanding and interpreting the war.³ But beyond their symbolic and ideological usefulness, soldiers' bodies were also *literally* useful. Splintered femurs could offer insight into the ways minié balls affected bone, and bits of necrosed bowel might carry lessons about the effects of diarrheal disease. As Brinton's assistant curator pointedly reminded the young private, the government, in the form of the Union army's Medical Department, was entitled to the bodies of its soldiers for as long as they served a purpose.

Generally, historians contend that, despite its morbidity, the Army Medical Museum's collection of military specimens and photographs was an important, necessary part of the progress of American medicine and an irreplaceable archive of Civil War history.⁴ Shauna Devine, for instance, interprets the reduction of a "soldier to his most useful parts" as evidence of the advance of scientific medicine toward today's clinical detachment and professionalism.⁵ This was undoubtedly true. Anatomical knowledge was a critical facet of the rise of professional medicine, and it helped to save lives. But this triumphal narrative glosses over the ethical questions inherent in the collection of human remains for study and display.

Much of the history of disability in the United States centers on the ways medical authorities used and abused disabled bodies.⁶ Soldiers' bodies differed from other disabled bodies; they were imbued with beliefs about manhood, duty, and honor; and their physical differences were typically newly formed. Even so, the creation of the Army Medical Museum should be understood within the larger history of medical authority and disability. I do not mean to cast the many physicians of the Army Medical Department (AMD) as one-dimensional cackling villains. Dedicated to serving sick and suffering soldiers, Union medical officers believed they had the good fortune to be part of advancing American medical science to benefit future patients. But just as the war machine needed bodies, medical progress required bodies (or at least *parts* of bodies) to move forward, and Union doctors had unprecedented access.

Informed consent was decades away from entering the medical lexicon during the Civil War. Yet historians agree that medical authorities overstepped their bounds at times during the nineteenth century, particularly in the maltreatment of the disabled and mentally ill and the use of black, Native American, and disabled bodies for dissection or medical research.⁷ All such "specimens," like the wounds and ailments of Union soldiers, were justified by their potential to advance scientific medicine and help to affirm professional physicians' authority. Doctors' and surgeons' power over the body was assumed. In addition, it was the official interpretation of the Army Medical Department that soldiers in particular had signed over their *bodies*, not just their lives, to the service of the United States government.[8] This contract afforded military medical authorities the right to collect amputated body parts, disinter corpses from graves, and display these items to the public through medical museums and exhibitions. Some men saw this arrangement as an extension of their duty. But for many outside the medical profession, the bleached bones, even when scrubbed of their names and histories, represented human suffering and the horrors of war.

Throughout the history of American warfare, the bodies of veterans and soldiers have been sites of symbolic potential. Veterans themselves sometimes embraced their status as living relics of the war. Brian Matthew Jordan relates the story of a former combatant who referred to himself as a "living monument of that late cruel and bloody Rebellion."[9] Many veterans took control of the ways in which the general public could use and interpret their disabled bodies, ensuring that the memory of the Civil War reflected their commitment to the Union cause. The idea that bodies could be monuments suggests that, in a sense, bodies did not belong to soldiers alone. Indeed, historian Lisa Herschbach argues that the physical sacrifices of the Civil War were understood within "an established Christian aesthetic linking individual injury to collective rejuvenation."[10] "Empty sleeves" belonged to the public at large and functioned as reminders of the won—or in the South, lost—cause.[11] Soldiers and veterans, in serving a cause bigger than themselves, were expected to transcend the individual. For disabled soldiers and their comrades, this meant subverting individual ownership of the body for the greater good as doctors seized body parts in the name of medical progress.

The Civil War came at an important juncture for American medicine. Before the war, the medical profession in the United States was fragmentary. Medical education lacked standardization, and no licensing system regulated the practices of individual doctors. In addition, the American Medical Association was only about ten years old. Of more concern were bitter contests over the place that science should assume in antebellum medicine. This struggle played out in division between "regulars," doctors who placed high value on scientific research and practices, and "irregulars," physicians who distrusted science and instead practiced homeopathy or botanic medicine. The divide between these camps dominated American medicine in the decades before and after Civil War, with particular concern over which group would become the dominant medical power.[12]

The tremendous need for surgeons during the war presented an opportunity for medical professionals. Both homeopaths and regulars attempted to join the ranks of the medical service, in part because they wanted to serve the Union cause, but also because it seemed clear that the faction that controlled the Army Medical Department could potentially control the American medical profession. Seeing the chance to destroy the competition and use the war to cement its position, the AMD set strict standards for physician enlistment to ensure that only well-qualified regulars won placements. Doctors seeking to serve were examined before a board of elite physicians. Those seeking regular army commissions were subjected to a multipart examination that included a written test, an essay, an oral examination, and several observations in surgeries, clinics, and autopsies. Because of these strict standards, by 1862, the department was populated with some of the best physicians in the United States. Its leadership ensured that military surgeons were not only talented and highly trained, but also enthusiastic about and committed to the advancement of medicine as a science and a profession.[13]

While the war offered the chance to establish medical authority, it also offered regulars the opportunity to advance the study of medicine. On May 21, 1862, only a few weeks after his appointment as surgeon general, Dr. William Hammond issued Circular No. 2 to the surgeons working beneath him in the AMD. Few of the department's actions did more to define the purpose of the Union's Civil War medical service. Circular No. 2 required military surgeons to "diligently collect and forward to the office of the Surgeon General all specimens of morbid anatomy, surgical or medical, which [might] be regarded as valuable; together with projectiles and foreign bodies removed; and such other matter as [might] prove of interest in the study of military medicine and surgery."[14] In other words, army surgeons were authorized and required to gather physical evidence of interesting cases—including bones, body parts, even entire cadavers—and forward them to the office of the surgeon general.

Only a few weeks later, Hammond issued Circular No. 5, which required Union army surgeons to send detailed reports of compelling cases to the surgeon general's office, and General Order 116, which called for the creation of a medical museum and laboratory for the study of the specimens.[15] With these orders, Surgeon General Hammond redefined the Army Medical Department, expanding its purpose to include the scientific advancement of American medicine. In addition, Hammond's measures gave medical doctors another level of authority. They now held sway not only over the bodies of the sick and wounded but also those of the dead.

To Hammond and his colleagues, the war presented a rare opportunity to learn from the human body. Medical use of the deceased body for dissection and autopsy was a deeply controversial topic in nineteenth-century America. Between 1785 and 1855, no less than seventeen "anatomy riots" and countless smaller conflicts erupted from outrage over the medical use of corpses.[16] Regular doctors believed their knowledge of anatomy set them apart from homeopaths, botanists, and midwives, and, importantly, the general public, who treated the deceased body with sentiment rather than scientific reason.[17] It was exactly this sentiment that made dissection so difficult. Families were reluctant to allow their loved ones' bodies on the autopsy table. Inspired by the 1832 British Anatomy Act, numerous states attempted to pass anatomy acts during the 1830s and 1840s. These measures would provide medical schools with the bodies of the indigent poor and prisoners for dissection. The idea was that those who had relied on public relief during their lifetimes would "pay back" their debts with their corpses. However, the public saw through the classist underpinnings of the acts and repeatedly rejected them. Those statutes that passed were often repealed after a short period due to powerful backlash from the public. New York State, for instance, tried four separate times to pass an anatomy act between 1830 and 1845—but every single bill died.[18]

The bodies of the dead held immense meaning for antebellum Americans, who loved sentimental poems, stories, and images depicting beautiful corpses. Antebellum mourning culture fixated on the peaceful and angelic nature of the deceased. A particularly iconic example of this notion is the death of Little Eva in *Uncle Tom's Cabin*; author Harriet Beecher Stowe describes the deceased child as having a "high celestial expression ... mingling rapture and repose."[19] According to Michael Sappol, antebellum Americans considered dissection akin to rape, a desecration of the body and violation of the beautiful death. Americans also feared death's potential to strip the body of its individuality, and they likewise took steps to prevent anonymity through memorialization. When loved ones were buried, they were given discrete spaces and personalized memorials. Dissection, like being buried in a mass grave or potter's field, meant that the body became "a collection of body parts and waste."[20] Drew Gilpin Faust argues that the body "represented the intrinsic selfhood and individuality of a particular human, and at the same time it incarnated the very humanness of that identity—the promise of eternal life that differentiates human remains from the carcasses of animals."[21] Stripping a body of its individual identity by breaking it down into so many parts was profoundly disturbing.

Because of the unpopularity of anatomy acts in the decades before the war, doctors and medical students were in constant contention for access to cadavers for hands-on training in human anatomy. Medical schools had to rely on executed criminals and bodies stolen from the grave. While the middle and upper classes could protect their dead from thieves with expensive coffins and gated cemeteries, poor and marginalized communities of the enslaved, free blacks, Native Americans, and the Irish could not, and so were the most likely targets for body snatchers.[22] For surgeons, then, the Civil War offered a perfect solution: they had fairly unlimited access to wounded bodies, offering them the opportunity to practice their skills and test treatment options.

If their patients died, surgeons had the prerogative to perform postmortem analyses and, under Circular No. 2, collect body parts for further study. Bodies were plentiful, and the war made it difficult for patients and families to object to their medical use. While surgeons were officers, most patients were enlisted men, which meant that they or their comrade advocates were often reticent to cross a superior officer by refusing a perceived order. Families were typically absent when a soldier died. They often did not receive notice of their loved one's death until days or weeks later, making it nearly impossible for them to protest. Even if someone did object, the circular gave Army Medical Department officials express authority to seize body parts as they saw fit, meaning that they weren't acting as body snatchers when they disinterred body parts. However, as we will see, not all agreed with this determination.[23]

The materials collected under Circular No. 2 and forwarded to the office of the surgeon general were used to fill the newly established Army Medical Museum. Surgeon-curator John Brinton, the museum's young, classically trained director, had earned a degree from the respected Jefferson Medical School in Philadelphia and completed advanced scientific medical and anatomical training in the best schools in Europe.[24] Surgeon General Howard directed Brinton to gather and arrange collected specimens into a "Military Medical Museum," to gather more specimens, and to report any military surgeons who neglected or refused to forward materials to the museum. Brinton was delighted with the assignment—his "whole heart" was in the museum, he later recalled. (Despite his penchant for preserving body parts, he did not mean this literally.) The surgeons of the Union army now had the opportunity to create their own "grand national cabinet" that would help to place the American medical profession on par with its more prestigious European counterparts. Medical colleges in Europe often had large anatomical collections.[25] Brinton believed that the "results of the surgery of this war would be preserved for all time, and the education of future generations of military surgeons would be greatly assisted."[26]

The growth of Brinton's museum relied not only on the cooperation of other military surgeons, but more specifically on the wounding and death of Union soldiers. "First of all," Brinton recalled, explaining the process by which the museum gathered its specimens, "the man had to be shot, or injured, to be taken to the hospital for examination, and in a case for operation, to be operated on." Then "the bones of a part removed" would be cleaned and stored in a barrel filled with alcohol, usually whiskey, or salt water.[27] When the barrel was sufficiently jammed with anatomical specimens, it would be shipped to Washington, where the parts would be cleaned, preserved, and mounted for display.

At times, particularly in the museum's first year, surgeons found it challenging to gather and prepare specimens. "In the case of field hospitals," Brinton noted, "after great battles, it was at first difficult to get our system to work." After large engagements, physicians and hospital staff were overwhelmed and overworked, and collecting samples for the museum was often impossible or impractical. So Brinton swooped in after these "great battles" to "overcome all these difficulties and to set an example," and he assumed the task himself. Visiting these hospitals gave him the chance to observe field surgeries. More importantly, he "had the opportunity of showing practically to the operating surgeons, and to their assistant staffs, what it was [the museum] really wanted."[28] Brinton's memoirs suggest that collection of specimens the museum "really wanted" was his true goal, not effectively treating the wounded soldiers. Brinton was truly committed to the museum. He even disinterred hastily buried bodies to gather discarded specimens. "Many and many a putrid heap have I dug out of trenches where they have been buried, in the supposition of an everlasting rest, and ghoul-like work I have done."[29] There was no everlasting rest in the march of medicine.

Brinton's frankness about exhuming "putrid heaps" stood in stark contrast to Victorian sentimentality regarding death and the sanctity of corpses. In his hands, the sacred bodies of military dead transformed into potential anatomical prizes for the Army Medical Museum. In one sense, Brinton's attitude toward specimens can be ascribed to developing clinical detachment, or the ability to maintain distance during difficult situations in order to remain professional. Before the Civil War, detachment was not necessarily part of a doctor's skill set. Many doctors worked in small towns with patients they knew personally, making detachment difficult, if not impossible, to cultivate. The Army Medical Department, however, made this skill a central part of its philosophy.[30] John Shaw Billings, longtime director of the library at the Army Medical Museum, insisted, "The emotional element does not enter into it at all." Once separated from its source, it didn't matter whether a specimen of stomach cancer was "from the body of Napoleon and not from an unknown soldier."[31] Achieving this level of detachment was a mark of professionalism. Yet, as anthropologist Simon Harrison suggests in his analysis of bone collectors, specimen gathering could become a quest or a hunt even for professional scientists and physicians. Rather than feeling clinical dispassion, collectors often recalled in their memoirs "daring escapades, their perseverance and dedication, and the difficulties, hardships and dangers they overcame for the sake of science."[32]

In his zeal, Brinton certainly exhibited the traits of an explorer. Collecting specimens was not a passive endeavor, and he engaged in a few daring escapades as he endeavored to secure his prize. In December 1862, Brinton rushed to Fredericksburg to assist field surgeons and seek out materials for the Army Medical Museum. Arriving before the battle had quite ended, he narrowly avoided becoming a specimen himself as Confederate batteries bombarded the town. When he learned that the Army of the Potomac planned to withdraw toward the banks of the Rappahannock River, Brinton and his assistant attempted to move their amassed specimens to safety. They came under fire as they approached the banks of the river. Relieved to have survived, Brinton's assistant, Dr. Moss, remarked, "What a blessed escape, for what a wretched ending it would have been to one's life, to have been swept into the river on an ignominious retreat, holding onto a bag of bones."[33] Moss and Brinton, managing to avoid both the whizzing minié balls and the rushing Rappahannock, safely delivered their collection to the museum.

Though the museum was initially created for use by doctors and surgeons practiced in the art of clinical detachment, it was also open to the general public. During the late eighteenth and early nineteenth centuries, such openness was common. As anatomical museums gained a reputation as cheap amusements, institutions began closing their doors to all but qualified medical professionals.[34] The Army Medical Museum, however, remained open to the general public. This decision owed at least in part to the museum's federal funding. But the museum's creators also wanted to demonstrate to the public the "scientific authority and social prominence of the orthodox physician" in the hope of exorcising the irregulars for good.[35] Even so, most visitors were drawn by the idea of glimpsing relics of the war.

Unlike physicians, who might value the anonymous scientific value of bones and specimens, most public visitors could not help meditating on the owners of the limbs the museum displayed. It was important for them to know whose body parts they were viewing. "When people come to the Army Medical Museum and ask where General Smith's brain . . . is, and are informed by the attendant that he does not know where it is, and is not even certain that it is in the collection, there are some expressions of disappointment," wrote Billings. The body parts of renowned generals were a big draw—Dan Sickles's amputated right leg, removed on the field at Gettysburg, was particularly popular. Though Sickles's leg and other famous body parts were major attractions, they weren't the only things the public hoped to see.[36] Many hoped and sometimes dreaded the thought of seeing their own body parts or those of a loved one. For this reason, John Billings argued, most of the specimens remained anonymous: "One would not like to have his or her father's skull displayed and labeled with his name, no matter how great or how infamous he may have been."[37] Displaying bones and bits of flesh without labels did not necessarily stop laypeople from contemplating whether a specimen was part of someone they loved.

Even if they were not labeled by name, most the of the bones in the museum were accompanied by a card supplying brief descriptions of the case. In her review of the museum, journalist Mary Clemmer Ames described "a piece of a human cranium, about the size of a silver dollar, cut from the head of a soldier wounded at Petersburg, Va., June 14, 1864."[38] The specimen's accompanying explanation provided a horrific description of a traumatic head wound. When admitted to the hospital in Washington, the anonymous soldier was unconscious and having seizures. Bloodletting did not calm him, so surgeons removed portions of his skull, likely relieving the pressure of brain swelling and allowing the man to regain consciousness. But the open wound became infected, and more of the skull had to be removed. When the soldier's injury finally began to heal, doctors considered the case a success: "The patient's mental faculties were impaired somewhat, the ward-physician thought, but not to a great extent."[39]

This anonymous skull fragment was a typical specimen, and in many ways, it exemplified the Army Medical Museum's use and exhibition of soldiers' body parts. Beyond the triumphant note that the patient had survived—not an achievement on the soldier's part, but one for the enterprising surgeon who had attended him—no regard was given to the remainder of the soldier's life. If he survived, a head wound that serious, especially one treated by removing a significant portion of the skull, would have significantly impacted his quality of life. Other soldiers who had portions of skull removed after a head wound experienced substantial aftereffects from their injuries. For instance, Pvt. James Duffy of the 116th Pennsylvania Volunteers was hit with a piece of shell at the Battle of Chancellorsville, but he survived the injury and the removal of fifteen shattered pieces of his skull. A pension examiner noted in 1867 that Duffy suffered fainting spells and periods of

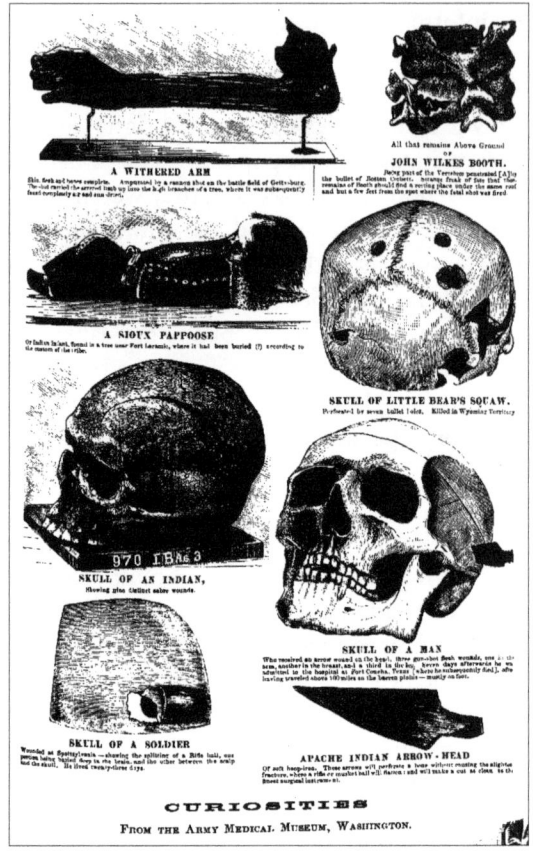

FIGURE 4. A selection of specimens at the Army Medical Museum in 1874. The described skull fragment appears at bottom left; another soldier's arm, voluntarily donated to the museum, is displayed at top left. These specimens are surrounded by the body parts and corpses of Native Americans who were disinterred or collected and displayed either without consent or with coerced consent. Mary Clemmer Ames, *Ten Years in Washington: Life and Scenes in the National Capital, As a Woman Sees Them* (Hartford: A. D. Worthington, 1873). Retrieved from the Library of Congress.

dizziness. In addition, he could not bear to be in the sun.[40] Alfred Green of the Seventy-Sixth Pennsylvania Volunteers was shot in the forehead at the Battle of Fort Wagner, South Carolina. When he arrived at a government hospital in Philadelphia several months later, he had portions of dead bone removed from the wound. After a short convalescence, Green was transferred to the Veteran Reserve (Invalid) Corps. In 1870, another pension examiner noted that Green "was subject to frequent and severe convulsions of an epileptic character, which occur on an average once a week, and last from one-half to six hours."[41]

An engraving depicting a handful of the museum's holdings accompanied Ames's description of the skull fragment. In the image, the remains of Native Americans, including the body of a mummified child, surrounded soldiers' skulls and arms. The Army Medical Museum, like many museums of the age, collected the remains of indigenous people. These remains were also collected in the name of science, albeit a very different type of science. The skulls of Native Americans were often used in the study of craniometry, which posited that racial hierarchies could be determined through the careful measurement of the human skull. According to craniometrists, the skulls of whites held larger brains and thus indicated a greater level of civilization, while black and Native American skulls held smaller brains, evidencing less evolutionary development.[42] Another journalist, Joanna Nicholls Kyle, wrote in *Godey's Magazine* in 1898, "In the gallery [of the museum] is a collection of three or four thousand Indian skulls of different tribes." Nearby, she added, "a long array of complete skeletons [were] suspended in a continuous glass case, [lining] the whole length of one side of the gallery-wall." The Medical Museum also showcased a collection of preserved Native American babies that would make visitors "gaze in wonder."[43]

The Army Medical Department intended that these collections be perceived differently. Both military and Native bodies forwarded scientific medicine, but the continued display of their bones was justified in different ways. Encasing bits of soldiers' bodies in glass was framed as a way of honoring the physical sacrifice of war. In contrast, the Medical Museum displayed Native American bodies as artifacts of natural history.[44] But the difference between honored soldiers and animallike Native people was not always so clear to patrons. In some cases, combatants' bodies were also described in relation to the natural world. Joanna Nicholls Kyle noted in 1898 that a display on veterinary surgery was located near a case of plaster casts of amputated limbs and soldiers' bullet-riddled bones, observing, "The horse is eminently man's close companion and friend in time of war."[45]

Race complicated matters further. Typically, black, white, and Native bodies were separated even in death, interred in segregated cemeteries. Confederate soldiers occasionally buried white officers—famously, Col. Robert Gould Shaw—with their black soldiers as an insult.[46] The Medical Museum displayed the remains of whites and Natives separately, but not far from one another. Whether certain bones belonged to white soldiers or indigenous peoples would not have been immediately apparent without their descriptive placards. Without the captions, the skulls in Ames's illustration just look like skulls—no racial difference is apparent. The museum organizers might have seen these collections as vastly different, but it was difficult for laypeople to grasp the ideological differences when the remains of so many animals, soldiers, and Native Americans commingled.[47] And though soldiers' and Native Americans' bodies were appropriated within different contexts, their combined presence within the Army Medical Museum spoke to medical authorities' power over vulnerable bodies.

When skull collectors gathered the remains of Native people, they had no need to justify their actions with ideological arguments. However, Army Medical Department surgeons sometimes had to defend gathering bits of dead soldiers when comrades or court-martial boards questioned their intentions. Military physicians often employed the powerful language of honor and duty to convince soldiers that relinquishing their body parts, or those of their friends, was part of their duty as citizen-soldiers. John Brinton crafted a compelling argument along these lines. Brinton's colleagues informed him of a soldier's unique leg wound, but he subsequently learned that the injured man had died before his leg could be amputated. The attending surgeons wanted to keep the young soldier's limb as a specimen for the Army Medical Museum. The man's friends refused this request and buried their dead comrade, leg and all.

Brinton was not easily dissuaded. He went to the dead soldier's friends and made his case: "[I] explained my object, dwelt upon the glory of a patriot having *part* of his body at least under the special guard of his country, spoke of the desire of the Surgeon-General to have that bone, with all such similar arguments I could adduce."[48] Brinton used a language of sacrifice that soldiers were steeped in. Their friend was a patriot who had made the ultimate sacrifice for his country. Now, Brinton argued, the country could repay its debt to the fallen soldier by displaying his leg at the Army Medical Museum. The limb would symbolize the sacrifices of the many soldiers who had lost their arms, legs, and lives in the Civil War.

The dead man's friends understood the subtext in Brinton's lofty assurances. Giving the limb to the museum was an extension of the dead man's duty as a soldier; just as he had offered his life for his country, he now had to offer his leg. "The comrades of the dead soldier solemnly decided that I should have that bone for the good of the country," Brinton recalled with satisfaction, "and in a body they marched out and dug up the body." The language of sacrifice left the slain man's friends with no choice. If they refused, they would not only defy a senior officer, but also prove themselves poor men who refused to serve their country in its need. As Brinton removed the dead soldier's leg, apparently right there at the graveside, one of the man's friends murmured, "John would have given it . . . himself, had he been able to express his opinion."[49]

While John's friends reluctantly complied with Brinton's request, other soldiers protested more vehemently against surgeons' appropriation of combatants' bodies. Just weeks before Surgeon General Hammond issued Circular No. 2, William H. D. Hatton, chaplain of the First Pennsylvania Rifles, told regimental commander George McCall about a horrific event he had witnessed on the Manassas battlefield. "Impelled by a sense of humanity, as well as a feeling of respect for the quiet repose of the sacred remains of the Patriot Dead," Hatton wrote, "I deem it my duty to lay before you a statement of facts."[50] The chaplain had witnessed Edward Donnelly, one of the surgeons of the Fifth Corps, stooping over the shallow improvised grave of Union soldiers hastily buried after the battle nearly a year previous. Donnelly was "rooting out the remains of one of those unfortunate men, who fell there and which was merely covered by the Rebels in the place where found."[51] The surgeon had already placed some leg bones into a bag, and he was in the process of separating the ankle and foot bones from the remaining flesh and clothing.

Disgusted, Hatton shouted at the surgeon, accusing him of "a second addition of the Rebel atrocities on the remains of [the Union] dead." Unmoved, Donnelly responded, "Every man has his peculiar taste in such matters." According to Hatton, Donnelly intended to send the bones as a "novelty" to a "New York museum." The chaplain assumed their destination was the popular if tawdry American Museum, operated by famed showman P. T. Barnum.[52] Hatton concluded his letter to General McCall by noting, "If such acts are to be perpetrated (as I learn they are every day by such men) unnoticed and unpunished by our Federal army, I think we need say no more about Rebel barbarism."[53]

General McCall immediately forwarded the matter to brigade commander John F. Reynolds. Appalled, Reynolds insisted that Donnelly either be immediately dismissed or brought before a court of inquiry to determine whether he had behaved improperly. During the inquiry, witnesses testified that Donnelly had not dug up the bones, but rather had collected them from where they had lain scattered on the ground, unburied. Testimony also emphasized Donnelly's passion for scientific medicine that gave him a great fondness for "relics." The case then revolved around the question of whether Donnelly had disinterred the bones, or whether he had simply collected them from the surface of the battlefield. The court of inquiry decided that a court-martial was warranted. Donnelly pled guilty to collecting the bones but denied desecrating any graves or intending to send the bones to a museum. He was found guilty, but the court added that his guilt had no "criminality" associated with it, and Donnelly was returned to active service.[54]

Hatton had reacted so vehemently to Donnelly's collecting because he believed the surgeon was gathering bones as trophies of the battle. Much trophy hunting during the Civil War focused on dropped weapons, spent bullets, and even parts of the natural environment, such as the trees at

Appomattox Court House. Even so, as in many previous and succeeding wars, it was not uncommon for civilians and soldiers themselves to gather body parts of the enemy dead as war prizes.[55] One Southern nurse recalled a fellow guest at a dinner party asking her to find the skull of a dead Yankee—the woman planned to keep knickknacks in it. A cavalryman from Virginia told his family that his brother was whittling a ring from the leg bone of a Union soldier. The collection of mementos from the dead, including hair jewelry, photographs, or paintings, was a key part of antebellum mourning culture, so gathering body parts was not entirely unprecedented. But trophy hunting took place outside the bounds of personal mourning, separating body parts from the memory of an individual deceased person. It also used those remains to flaunt, humiliate, and terrify.[56] To Hatton, Donnelly's collections from the dead bodies of First Bull Run reduced the remains to so many useful bones and violated their sacred nature.

Donnelly's case shows just how bitterly contested the idea of gathering specimens from battlegrounds could be. Donnelly maintained that he only gathered the bones out of a professional desire to learn. To his mind, this carried no disrespect or offense to the dead. "Mr. Hatton's letter," Donnelly declared in his written statement to the court of inquiry, "had by a singular perversion of language magnified the simple act of my picking up a few bones into a great crime." Donnelly also vehemently denied that the bones were destined for P. T. Barnum's museum. To display the bodies of war dead in such a public museum, he stated, "would have been contrary to the characteristic reverence my countrymen have for the remains of the dead; it would have been contrary to the teachings of my Holy Church!"[57] As a medical professional, Donnelly found no moral quandary in keeping the bones for his own use. Hatton and Reynolds, on the other hand, clearly considered his actions enough of an insult to the anonymous Union dead to pursue a court-martial. Hatton deemed the act of collecting soldiers' remains an "act of inhuman vandalism" and a "disgrace to our army and nation."[58] Regardless of whether Army Medical Department surgeons maintained that such collections of human remains were for scientific purposes with no "emotional element," those outside the medical establishment clearly considered such actions desecrations whether the bodies were properly buried or not.

Donnelly was not the only surgeon of the AMD that came under scrutiny for attempting to gather anatomical specimens. George Potts, the white regimental surgeon of the Twenty-Third United States Colored Troops (USCT), was court-martialed when other members of his regiment discovered his activities late on the night of March 21, 1865. Earlier that day,

Pvt. Benjamin Anderson, a former slave who had joined the regiment in 1864, had suddenly and mysteriously dropped dead as he stepped out of his tent.[59] Dr. Potts ordered that Anderson's body be moved to the medical tent for an autopsy. Anderson's naked corpse remained in the tent for some four hours until Potts was ready to begin. When he finally commenced work, Potts removed Anderson's heart without closing off the surrounding blood vessels, which resulted in profuse bleeding that rendered the hospital tent "perfectly horrible." Undisturbed, the doctor explored the rest of Anderson's flayed body, eventually discovering several abnormalities in the abdominal organs. He turned to his assistant, Dr. Bethel, and said he "thought they were perfect curiosities," which he would send "to the Surgeon General for microscopic examination and for the medical museum in Washington, DC."[60] He requested that Bethel scrounge up some whiskey for storing the organs.

By that time, Dr. Potts was growing tired, as it was "near midnight and raining, and the floor of the tent was flooded and slippery." Before quitting for the evening, he decapitated Anderson, hoping to remove the man's brain in the morning. After closing the body, Potts apparently worried that the presence of a headless corpse would arouse concern. He placed a glass bottle wrapped in rags where Anderson's head might otherwise have been, then sewed a blanket closed around the body. Potts placed Anderson's organs and head in a box, wrapped it in canvas, and tucked it under the table. When he returned to his tent for the night, he began worrying that a stray dog might find the aforementioned body parts, so he sneaked back into the hospital tent at about 2:00 a.m. and brought the box of viscera back to his own quarters. Too curious about Anderson's head to sleep, Potts began his examination. Lt. Col. Marshall Dempsey entered the doctor's tent just as he was peeling back Anderson's scalp and preparing to open his skull with a bone saw. The horrified commanding officer demanded that Potts stop his work immediately and turn over the rest of Anderson's body parts. Disappointed to lose an impressive specimen for the museum, Potts begrudgingly complied.[61]

The resulting court-martial, like Dr. Donnelly's, centered on conflicting beliefs about the bodies of dead soldiers. To Potts, the matter seemed entirely routine. Benjamin Anderson was not only a dead soldier with interesting internal organs, he was a black soldier who had died in the custody of white medical officers—which only made him more accessible to the medical authority. Conducting a postmortem seemed entirely natural to Potts. While it was very difficult for doctors and medical students to gain access to white bodies for dissection or experimentation, it was fairly easy to obtain black bodies, especially those of the enslaved. Bondsmen and bondswomen were routinely subjected to medical experimentations and procedures without their consent. Slaves' corpses were often seized or disinterred for use in anatomy laboratories in the South's medical schools.[62] J. Marion Sims, celebrated as the "father of modern gynecology," performed numerous nonconsensual surgeries and experiments on enslaved men and women. He perfected his most famous surgical innovation, the repair of vesico-vaginal fistulas, on the bodies of slave women whose owners had volunteered them for his study. Sims and his students operated on a woman named Anarcha thirty times in five years without her consent.[63]

Blacks' bodies were also more easily procured for dissection. Although enslaved people believed strongly that postmortem destruction of the body jeopardized the deceased's ability to rest in peace, they rarely had the ability to refuse autopsies. That decision fell to their masters.[64] It was also common for medical schools and practitioners to receive the bodies of executed blacks, and to disinter bodies from black cemeteries. The pervasive fear that doctors would snatch black bodies led to the "night doctor" character in southern African American folklore. This physician or grave robber seized black bodies to use in gruesome medical experimentation. As Potts demonstrates, these bogeymen were not without foundation.[65]

The commanding officers and soldiers of the Twenty-Third USCT found the autopsy of Anderson inappropriate and horrifying. Even young Dr. Bethel was offended, and he acted as the key witness in the resulting court-martial. The usefulness of Anderson's organs to the betterment of science mattered little to the men who had served alongside him. To them, decapitating their comrade was nothing more than an act of depraved desecration. The skull and brain were not interesting specimens, but the head of their friend. If action wasn't taken against Potts, Dempsey noted, it would "demoralize the troops and destroy all confidence and discipline."[66] The lieutenant colonel doubtless had another worry. Potts's apparent confirmation of fears that white fdoctors would mutilate black bodies could corrode the men's trust in Dempsey's and other white officers' leadership.

William Conover, medical director of the Twenty-Fifth Corps, succinctly expressed the feelings of the rest of the regiment: "This case was not a Post Mortem examination, or a dissection: it was a mutilation of the body not justifiable."[67] While Conover agreed that autopsies and dissections could be performed on surgeons' best judgment, they had to be done with a sense of propriety, even on the field of battle and even on a black soldier. Thus he recommended that Potts be cashiered. Despite his attempts to defend himself by claiming he was only trying to learn from Anderson's body and gather specimens for the museum, Potts was ordered dishonorably discharged "for unjustifiably mutilating the body of a dead soldier, in the presence of the enlisted men of the command."[68]

Potts's trial and conviction showed the limits to medical power. Had the surgeon discreetly autopsied Anderson in the light of day and shipped his organs to the Medical Museum, he likely would have avoided a court-martial board. Edward Donnelly could make the case that his acquisition of dry, disarticulated bones was scientifically warranted. The ankle and foot bone were devoid of any individuality. In his bloody midnight mutilation of Private Anderson, Potts tried and failed to turn a man into an object right in his own camp: the blood and viscera on the doctor's hands silently testified to the soldier's humanity.

After the war, the holdings of the Army Medical Museum continued to elicit mixed reactions from patrons, civilians and veterans alike. According to its employees, the museum was a popular destination for visitors to Washington, DC, an estimated six thousand of whom had toured the collections by 1867.[69] It's not clear how many within that number were laypeople. What is apparent is the fact that some outside the medical profession did not consider the museum a happy destination. In 1873, journalist Louis Bagger suggested that the institution was the least visited one in Washington. In her detailed 1874 review of the museum, Mary Clemmer Ames suggested that while some of the displays might be interesting, perhaps even beautiful, the suffering the specimens portrayed was more than most people could bear. "It cannot fail to be one of the most absorbing spots on earth to the student of surgery or medicine," she admitted, "but to the unscientific mind, especially to one still aching with memories of the war, it must ever remain a museum of horrors."[70]

An unnamed correspondent to the *Washington Star* agreed with Ames's estimation a decade later. The descriptions of the museum's holdings in the newspaper differ markedly from the clinical descriptions offered by John Shaw Billings and John Brinton. Instead, the journalist emphasized the brutality of both warfare and surgeons' cures.

> One case is devoted to arms and legs that have been amputated, and show how nice and slick the surgeon's knife and saw went through. Some are lacerated and torn to pieces by gunshot wounds. Most of the exhibits are the scraps of men picked up off the battlefield. One heart has two big ... bullets embedded in it.... There are all sorts of human bones shattered by shot and shell. Skulls with great big lead balls sticking in them; big bones with

fragments of iron shells crushing them into powder; joints broken apart by musket balls, there are skulls, ribs, legs and arms, shattered and shivered by all sorts of missiles of war, and in some cases the lead and bone have become welded together. There are over 9,000 specimens of bones fractured in curious ways by shot.[71]

For the reporter from the *Washington Star*, the bits of human bodies displayed at the museum represented the horrors of battle: bones were "lacerated," "torn," "shattered," "shivered," and "crushed" by the missiles of war. Curator J. J. Woodward's comments stand in stark contrast; he referred to bones as "osseous specimens" that were "preserved dry, neatly cleaned," and "mounted on little black stands."[72] Just as the Army Medical Museum cleaned soldiers' bones of their human flesh, they tried—not entirely successfully—to clean them of their human pain and suffering.

For some veterans, the museum's collections seemed to hold further evidence for old soldiers' calls for government support. Henry Van Ness Boynton, a Washington correspondent for the *Cincinnati Gazette* who was himself a wounded former Union officer, pointed to the tension between the medical and sentimental reactions to scientific renderings of the war's toll. A report on the museum and preliminary reports of casualty numbers prepared by the AMD in 1866 included this data. "These are the scientific facts which our armies have set forth in blood and suffering," Boynton wrote at the close of the otherwise dry article, asking, "How much of it is the country willing to forgive? How much of it shall politicians be allowed to cast aside as nothing worth?"[73] The colorless statistics of specimens in the museum and numbers of casualties represented more than just "the history of the care for the sick and wounded." This information instead represented the immense debt the North owed its veterans. These were scientific facts, Boynton admitted, but they were facts borne of human suffering.

Boynton's closing questions point to the larger issues those many bodily specimens called forth. When confronted with the physical ramifications of the war's brutality, could, or perhaps *should*, the citizens and leaders of the North be quick to forgive the newly reunited South? To Boynton, the remains that the curators of the Army Medical Museum worked so hard to reduce to their essential, medical nature instead carried great political significance. Each specimen taken from the body of a wounded Union soldier represented the South's treachery.

Despite its attempts to recast the bones of the Civil War dead as a part of the march of scientific progress, the Army Medical Department could never entirely separate the person from the body. The bones of soldiers, however dry, held complex meanings for those who viewed them. Boynton interpreted the "scientific facts" of the casualty numbers as evidence of Confederate barbarity. For her part, Mary Clemmer Ames saw bones as evidence of the great trauma of the war, each one symbolizing a loved one's grief. To the soldiers and officers of the Twenty-Third USCT, the autopsy of Benjamin Anderson was not part of scientific medicine's progress. It was an inexcusable desecration of human remains, another in a long line of medical abuses of black bodies. John Brinton boasted of the many impressive specimens he gathered for the museum, while other surgeons found themselves accused of grave robbing by those outside the medical professions. As hard as the doctors of the Medical Museum worked to separate the "emotional" element from the scientific, to soldiers and the public, bones were intrinsically tied to human bodies that had been stripped of their individual human identities.

Dead and disabled bodies have long come under the authority of doctors and surgeons claiming them as part of the materia medica of American scientific medicine. The physicians of the Army Medical Department and the curators of its museum exercised enormous power over the bodies of Union soldiers at their most vulnerable. To supply the Army Medical Museum with specimens that might educate future physicians and preserve Civil War medical history, Union doctors turned the bodies of soldiers into government property. Having bits of one's body preserved, these professionals argued, was another extension of a man's patriotic duty. Such efforts helped to cement the ascendancy of American scientific medicine, but that accomplishment raised difficult questions about medical power, consent, and soldiers' bodies. The Army Medical Department tried to frame the collection of white soldiers' bodies as a tribute to patriotic sacrifice and therefore different from the collection of other bodies. Yet soldiers and civilians did not always accept this interpretation. Truly, as John Brinton noted, dry bones were seen from different points of view.

In 1892, the Army Medical Museum took ownership of yet another bone—a hip bone plucked from the corpse of Maj. Gen. Henry A. Barnum. The bone was the last physical proof of Barnum's war trauma, a perforating gunshot wound that remained open and draining for thirty years. In life, the injury was easily hidden under his clothing; in death, this private wound was made publicly available. While opinions were divided about whether preserved body parts were an appropriate way to derive meaning from the war, nearly all postwar Americans agreed that the bodies of disabled soldiers were cultural touchstones. The image of the visibly disabled veteran became so ubiquitous as to become a trope—the "empty sleeve." The postwar public wanted to see and contemplate wooden legs and empty sleeves in order to help process the meanings of the war. But for veterans like Barnum, who bore wounds inaccessible to a stranger's gaze, the public's desire to investigate, verify, and contemplate wartime disability had complicated and sometimes emasculating consequences.

CHAPTER 4

The Disabled Lion of Union

On the night of June 17, 1864, Col. Joshua Lawrence Chamberlain walked anxiously among his sleeping soldiers. They were outside of Petersburg, Virginia, preparing for an attack against the Confederate city's fortifications. Something was bothering the colonel. He was no stranger to warfare—he had been in the hardest of the fights at Fredericksburg and Gettysburg—but something about this place felt different. "I had a strange feeling that evening, [a] premonition of coming ill," Chamberlain later wrote. "A dark shadow seemed to brood over me, dark wings folding as it were . . . and wrapping me in their embrace."[1] His unnerving premonition proved true. The next afternoon, Chamberlain led his men in an attack against Rives's Salient on the heavily fortified Confederate Dimmock Line around Petersburg. The fight quickly intensified. As the troops moved forward, they encountered wet, marshy land that would be difficult to cross. Chamberlain lifted his sword in one hand and the flag bearing the Maltese cross of the Fifth Corps in the other, using them to motion his men to the left. As he held the flag and sabre aloft, a minié ball smashed into his hip. It traveled through his right hip to the left, crushing his bones and cutting into his bladder and urethra. Blood pooled around his feet. Stunned, he braced himself with the flag and sword as his men passed, then the loss of blood brought him to his knees.

The next hours were surreal. Chamberlain remained aware of the clamor of battle, but his thoughts wandered toward his own bloody presence on the ground: "I lay now straight out on my back, too weak to move a limb; the blood forming a pool, under and around me—more blood than the books allow a man. I had not much pain. It was more a stunning blow, a

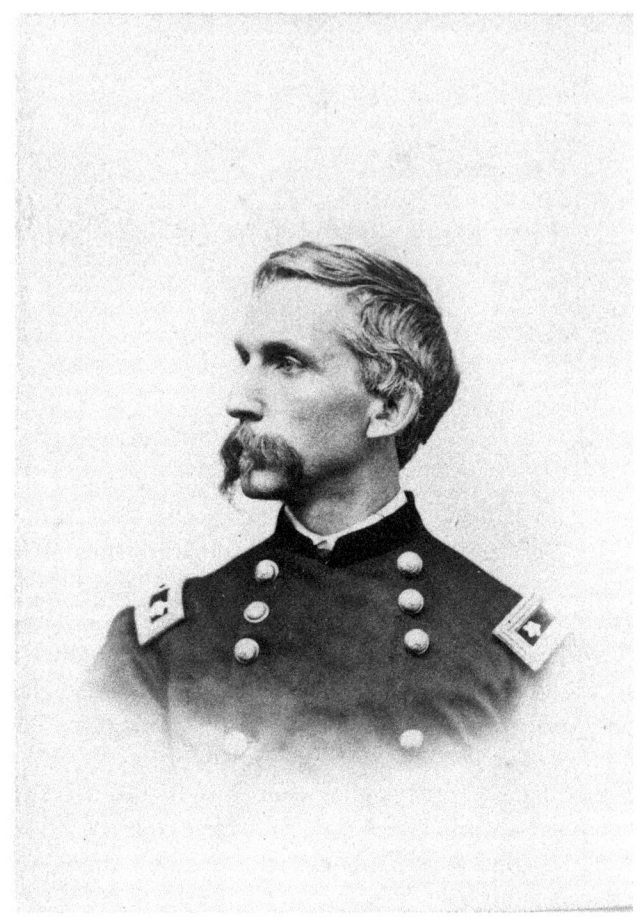

FIGURE 5. Bvt. Maj. Gen. Joshua Lawrence Chamberlain. Local Call Number M27, Bowdoin College Archives, Brunswick, ME.

kind of dull tension, my teeth shut sharp together hard, like lock-jaw. So I lay looking, thinking, sinking, the tornado tearing over and around. Dull hoarse faint cries in the low air: hisses, spatters, thuds, thunderbolts mingling earth and sky, and I moistening the little space of mother-earth for a cabbage-garden for some poor fellow, black or white, unthinking, unknowing."[2] Decades later, he would remember thinking of his mother as the life drained out of him.[3]

Chamberlain was removed to the division hospital, where surgeons explored the wound, which was too wide for standard surgical probes, with a ramrod. They were able to locate and cut out the ball, but little else could be done. Determined to accept the inevitable, Chamberlain asked the surgeons to leave him and put their efforts toward the other wounded men filling the hospital. The surgeons agreed. He wrote a bloodied last letter to his wife and lay back to wait for the end.[4]

But the end never came. Chamberlain survived that long night, though it seemed impossible even to him: "I never dreamed what pain could be and not kill a man outright."[5] When it seemed he might have a fighting chance, the surgeons attempted to correct some of the damage to his urethra. They managed to keep Chamberlain alive long enough to be transferred to the Annapolis Naval Hospital, where he could undergo more surgery. "For two months," he later recalled, he was "wrestling at the gates of death," enduring "convulsions, death-chills, lashings, despairing surgeons, waiting embalmers." But he survived. "Through this valley of the shadow death—in five months back at the front with my men!"[6] Chamberlain served out the remaining year of the war, was promoted twice for bravery, and left the army in 1865 as a brevet major general.

When Chamberlain returned to civilian life at the war's end, he seemed the embodiment of the ideal citizen-soldier—a charming, handsome war hero who had sacrificed but remained dedicated to cause and country. During his three years in the army, Chamberlain played a critical role in numerous battles. Though wounded six times and seriously ill twice, he returned quickly to the field each time and rose through the ranks. After the war, he leveraged his military reputation to win four years as the governor of Maine, then twelve years as the president of Bowdoin College. Adored among veterans, Chamberlain wrote extensively about the war and regularly served as a featured speaker at commemorations and encampments. The general's public image, however, concealed a more private dimension of his life.

Hidden beneath his blue uniform and fine suits, the wound from Petersburg quietly tortured Chamberlain. Because of the damage to his urethra, he had temporarily required a catheter after he was wounded. Friction from the catheter had created a fistula near the base of his penis that never healed.[7] It leaked urine and left him susceptible to chronic bladder and testicular infections that caused him, in his own words, "unspeakable agony."[8] A surgery in 1883 attempted to close the fistula. Chamberlain barely survived, and his symptoms—including the fistula—soon returned. Over the next thirty years, recurring infections plagued the general's self-described "weak spot," often incapacitating him.[9] A pension examiner noted in 1893 that painful adherent scars restricted Chamberlain's mobility. His testicles were permanently and painfully enlarged, and his penis was nonfunctioning.[10] When he died in 1914, it was of an infection of the old wound. Chamberlain was a casualty of war—it just had taken him fifty years to die.[11]

Studying Joshua Lawrence Chamberlain offers a rich opportunity to better understand Civil War disability. By situating him as a disabled person, it becomes apparent that the war's toll on bodies was more pervasive, persistent, and nuanced than historians often suggest. Chamberlain embodies Douglas Baynton's famous observation that disability is everywhere once you look for it, suggesting that a significant portion of Civil War disability has been hiding in plain sight.[12] In recent years, Civil War historians have had many fruitful debates over whether disabled veterans faced bitterness and defeat or had successful, well-adjusted postwar lives. Chamberlain's life demonstrates that for many the reality lay somewhere in the middle.[13] His experience was one of apparent contradictions; he was an ideal specimen of martial masculinity that was physically emasculated. He possessed some power over his public image and none over his pain or his pension. He wrote extensively about the glory of the won cause while searching for his own body's role in it. Chamberlain's example shows us that rather than falling into two opposing camps, disabled veterans actually occupied a liminal space, moving closer to one pole and then the other as their health, luck, and emotional state changed.

It has been possible to see Chamberlain as nondisabled because his wounds were not visually obvious. Nonvisible disabilities—wounds that were easily concealed under clothing or had no visual component, such as chronic illness or psychological trauma—accounted for the majority of Civil War wounds. Amputations were, and are, the disabilities most commonly associated with the war. Indeed, nearly all that has been written on Civil War disability has focused almost exclusively on amputees. Yet despite their outsize presence in the culture, amputees made up only a small percentage of disabled Union veterans. According to Theda Skocpol, 281,881 Union soldiers were wounded and survived the war. Of that number, only 20,802, or roughly 7 percent, were amputees.[14]

Though they may have been more common, nonvisible disabilities could also be more disconcerting for able-bodied Americans. These traumas offered few or no cues to differentiate the disabled from the nondisabled. As disability scholar N. Ann Davis argues, able-bodied people assume clear differences between their own bodies and the bodies of disabled people and thus question the legitimacy of disabilities that are not obvious. Nonvisibly disabled people must publicly disclose their disabilities in order to receive recognition. But when they do so, they are then subject to greater scrutiny and more frequently accused of fraud or malingering.[15] In the Civil War era, amputations were publicly viewed and contemplated, and as Frances Clarke notes, they "confirmed [veterans'] service and demanded acknowledgement and grateful remembrance."[16] The Northern public used imagery of disabled veterans as shorthand to signify the national suffering of the Civil War. These images almost always depicted an amputee, imbuing amputation with a cultural cachet other impairments lacked.[17] Men like Chamberlain did not see bodies like their own in the public dialogue on wartime disability. In order to claim their status as wounded veterans and obtain governmental support, men like Chamberlain had to publicly expose their infirmities in ways that challenged their manhood and resulted in humiliation.

Another consequence of the assumed significant differences between disabled and nondisabled bodies is that disability disappeared from the record. Because his wound was easily concealed, Chamberlain passed as able-bodied in most situations; as a result, he continues to pass as able-bodied in the historical narrative. Passing is a multifaceted phenomenon involving more than just concealing or revealing an impairment. Disability historian Michael Rembis points out that passing relies on how well one can adhere to societal norms of gender, race, behavior, and appearance.[18] While disability was often an experience in powerlessness, Chamberlain's identity as a middle-class white man and war hero afforded him at least the ability to control his image. Chamberlain did not (and could not) always conceal the effects of his wound. Yet he could mask the wound by adhering to able-bodied and masculine codes of behavior. Interpreting passing as evidence that veterans triumphed over disability falls into the overcoming narrative, a rejected interpretive mode that takes success as evidence that a person has transcended impairment.[19] Equating success with overcoming suggests that disability and achievement are mutually exclusive. It's also impossible: regardless of satisfaction, or inclusion, or attainment, the impairment is always present. Chamberlain's example serves as a reminder that many Civil War veterans experienced what Rembis refers to as a kind of disability double consciousness. The general lived as both a war hero and an emasculated cripple.[20]

Joshua Lawrence Chamberlain wrote about the war at great length as he aged, laboring over speeches and articles and manuscripts that might capture the essence of the most monumental event of his life. He wrote about the deaths of his men on Little Round Top, mourning the "manly resolution, heroic self-giving, divine reconciliation" of the young corpses, and honoring the suffering of the wounded.[21] *The Passing of the Armies*, Chamberlain's memoir of the last days of the war, meditates often, in his typically baroque style, on the meanings and costs of the war. Yet passages speculating on the meaning of sacrifice frequently use third person or plurals, prioritizing the abstract and obscuring the personal.[22] Chamberlain never described his own disability as a patriotic sacrifice. Rather, the near-fatal wound appeared more like an old and bitter enemy. For example, an unpublished 1899 manuscript describing Chamberlain's experience at Petersburg is suffused with a sense of dread. On the night before his charge at Rives's Salient, Chamberlain felt so assured of impending ill that he went so far as to bid farewell to division commander Gen. Charles Griffin. Much to Griffin's puzzled exasperation, Chamberlain predicted his own death the next day. "I had not the habit of taking a dark view of things," Chamberlain wrote. "[I was typically] resolved and ready to meet my fate, meaning to face it, and not flinch." Even so, he recalled that the night before the battle, a feeling of foreboding settled on him and "became oppressive, unbearable."[23] It's very possible that Chamberlain embellished his memories to create a more compelling drama, but it's telling that he chose to paint an ominous scene rather than emphasize his willingness to die. Perhaps three decades of pain darkened his memory.

Letters dating from the first months after his injury indicate that Chamberlain thought about his situation in grim terms. In January 1865, he received a leave from the army to undergo the first of three surgeries on his wound. The pause in military service provided him time and space to contemplate the future. Chamberlain's family hoped that the painful procedure would finally convince him to leave the army, but he soon announced that he would return to the front upon recovery. His mother, Sarah Chamberlain, unhappily argued that he had "done & suffered & won laurels enough in this war to satisfy the most ambitious."[24] Chamberlain disagreed. "Not all the titles that can be given or won would tempt me to hazard the happiness and welfare of my dear ones at home," he assured her. Titles and honors would be worthless to him anyway, he added, stating, "These terrible wounds ... must cast a shadow over the remainder of my days, even though I should apparently recover."[25] Chamberlain understood that although he had survived, his life would be significantly different. He described his wound not as necessary or honorable, but rather as "terrible," a trauma that would darken his future. Leaving the army would not change that. "It is a time when every man must stand by his guns," he later explained to his father. "And I am not scared or hurt enough to be willing to face the rear when other men are marching to the front."[26] Throughout his life, Chamberlain's private discussions of his wound in correspondence remained pragmatic and ambivalent.

Chamberlain was right to believe that the wound would have lasting repercussions. Before the Civil War, urological war injuries were often considered fatal and left untreated. By the latter years of the war, soldiers had a good chance of surviving such trauma if they could avoid secondary infection. Although soldiers survived in greater numbers, the aftereffects of their injuries haunted them. Damage to the pelvic bones impeded motion and caused chronic pain even when healed. Bladder wounds permanently affected bladder function and could cause persistent fistulas and recurrent cystitis. Wounds to the penis and testes often required amputation of the genitals. Even when these organs were saved, such wounds were often followed by depression and a sense of a "loss of virile power."[27] Urethral wounds like Chamberlain's were particularly difficult to repair, and they resulted in lifelong complications including painful, difficult, or uncontrolled urination. According to urologic surgeon Harry Herr, "one of every four survivors of urethral injuries required insertion of a catheter to evacuate urine, lived with an indwelling catheter, or wore other cumbersome collecting devices."[28]

Those who did not require or use catheters often lived with persistent urethral fistulas and urinary incontinence. According to pension examiners, one veteran suffered from a "deep-seated urethra-perineal fistula" accompanied by "loss of erectile power of the penis, with partial destruction of the left testis, and deformity of the scrotum." The man was incontinent, and this condition caused chronic skin irritation that, the examiners made sure to note, gave "rise to an exceedingly offensive odor." Another young man who was shot in the scrotum "suffered persistent urethral fistula, incontinence of urine, severe pain on exercise, and 'occasional discharges of matter from urethra and rectum.'"[29] Incontinence, of course, was not the only consequence of these disabilities. Men with urethral injuries faced the social ramifications of leaking urine, not to mention constant pain and recurrent infections. Perhaps the most devastating consequence of these wounds, however, was the loss or impairment of sexual function. For young men, the inability to have an intimate relationship or father children must have been emasculating. Thus the physical and emotional ramifications of such wounds were often kept deeply private.

Chamberlain's injury had similar complications. The entrance and exit wounds of the bullet had left adherent scars on each hip that made walking difficult and painful. He was unable to urinate in a typical way because of damage to his urethra from the original wound, prolonged catheterization, and multiple surgeries. Urine voided through a fistula in the base of his penis. The fistula would have leaked urine often, leading to chronic cystitis. Heavy surgical scarring on Chamberlain's perineum, reminders of procedures with good intentions and unfortunate outcomes, left the region highly sensitive. His prostate had atrophied, his penis was nonfunctioning,

78 Chapter 4

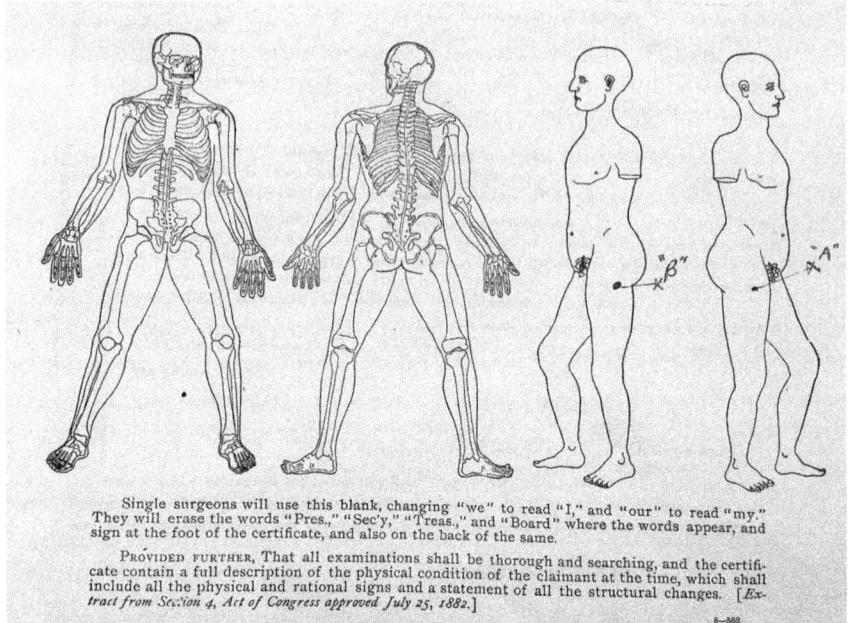

FIGURE 6. Surgeon's notations of entry and exit wounds on Chamberlain's hip. Surgeon's Certificate, 1893. Joshua Lawrence Chamberlain Military Pension Records, certificate 96,956, National Archives and Records Administration, National Archives Building, Washington, DC.

and his testicles were painfully inflamed from recurring bouts of orchitis and epididymitis.[30]

Despite chronic pain and recurring illness, Chamberlain was committed to appearing and acting as able-bodied as possible. He lived with the pain and relied on sheer willpower to continue working. His strict work ethic, coupled with a body that appeared outwardly whole and healthy, deflected attention away from his disability. His wounding was far from a secret—it had been covered in Northern newspapers—but Chamberlain worked hard to craft a public persona that proved him as capable and hardworking as ever. Just five months after he was shot, Chamberlain was back at the head of his brigade. He had difficulty walking and could not get into a saddle without help, but he assured his family in letters that he was "managing to do full duty without much injury, & not a great deal of suffering." Still, he admitted he did not feel "right yet."[31] While visiting camp in 1865, Chamberlain's father-in-law, Rev. George Adams, noted in his journal that Chamberlain was "pretty miserable but constantly working." Dr. DeWitt, head surgeon of the division, remarked to Adams that he "never saw a man who would continue working so when really unfit to move."[32]

When Chamberlain returned home at the war's end, the wound complicated his daily life, making it difficult to eat or sleep well. Although he had a desk chair made to accommodate his painful hips and groin, he was known to work while reclining on a sofa in his office when he could no longer sit upright.[33] His attempts to work as hard and as long as possible in spite of his health routinely left him sick and exhausted. Jenny Abbott, a family friend and a wheelchair user, chastised him for pushing his body too hard while governor. Few of Chamberlain's friends prodded him about his health like Abbott, who suffered long stretches of ill health and had no compunction in drawing comparisons between his disability and her own. In May 1872, when Chamberlain assured her that he was recuperating from another illness at his summer home in Maine and spending time on his new boat, Abbott responded, "Oh, let him [the doctor] help you, dear friend. I know the case is beyond the cure of the yacht."[34] She urged him to seek more medical wisdom, although thus far doctors had not provided him much relief. "When I recall all that you have triumphed over, I cannot feel that there is not still a great possibility of restoration to comfortable health. But it cannot come by unaided nature. . . . Only think for a little what it would be to have that dreadful wound put in a healthy condition!" Abbott assured Chamberlain that she understood what this meant. "Please, please, listen to me!" she pleaded in 1868. "You have borne for four years this cross—I for fourteen have borne a similar one and I know time does not make it easier."[35] We do not have Chamberlain's reply to her plea, but we do know that he did not relax his demanding schedule and resisted medical intervention except when absolutely necessary.

The complications of the wound sent reverberations through Chamberlain's marriage. Many tender letters between Chamberlain and his wife, Fanny, reveal the couple's loving physical relationship prior to his wounding. In their courtship, Chamberlain wrote frankly about his desire for Fanny. They discussed how they might time their first child, as well as how they might prevent pregnancies before the time was right.[36] Chamberlain's wartime letters make his attraction to his wife clear. "How happy I should be with my darling here for a little while just to enjoy this with me," he wrote to Fanny in late July 1863. He was still reeling from Gettysburg, and he teased Fanny that this fact was making him a bit forward. "You know I am not well yet that will account for my slight unsoundness of mind in a remark I just made to Col. Rice about a sweet smiling valley between the soft blue hills—'It is a vale of love, between the breasts of the Mountain.' Shall I be forgiven? and yet I half believe I should have said it to you, if you had been here—a soldier is bold, you know."[37]

But Joshua and Fanny's relationship grew strained when he returned home. His wound's role in the souring of their marriage is difficult to parse. Unsurprisingly, the couple's correspondence offers no clues as to their sexual relationship after the war, but modern urologists who have reviewed Chamberlain's pension and medical files conjecture that he would have found typical sexual function difficult if not impossible. In 1893, a surgeon reported to the pension board that Chamberlain's penis was nonfunctioning. Indeed, he and Fanny did not have any more children. However, while Fanny was forty years old in 1865, it was not uncommon for women of the era to conceive into their forties. It seems reasonable to speculate that the genital wound strained a relationship that the stressful war years and Chamberlain's immediate dive into work, travel, and politics had already made vulnerable.[38] In November 1868, simmering tensions came to a crisis. After Chamberlain, then the governor, had left Brunswick to return to Augusta, Fanny informed several acquaintances that he had physically and verbally abused her and denied her a divorce. Exhausted, unwell, and alone, Chamberlain had just arrived at the governor's residence and was attempting to sleep when an aide notified him of Fanny's accusations. Chamberlain was already in the midst of two of the major crises of his governorship, with furor rising over Maine's use of capital punishment and its stance on temperance, but the charge of marital mistreatment was far more upsetting.[39]

The incident was not the first time that the Chamberlains' marriage was shaken or that Fanny had discussed their relationship problems publicly. In his letter responding to her accusations, Chamberlain indicated that his wife's tendency to discuss their marriage with others had caused an ongoing disagreement between them, but one that he had, until recently, considered resolved. The couple had talked about the issue, and Fanny had apparently agreed to stop revealing their problems to others. Chamberlain seemed surprised she had gone back on her word. Now she was making their private troubles public once again. "Ms. Corlender it seems," Chamberlain wrote to Fanny, "is freely telling people that 'you told her (& Mrs. Dunning also as well as everybody else) that I stressed you beyond endurance, pulling your hair, striking, beating, & otherwise personally maltreating you, & that you were gathering up everything you could find against me to sue for divorce.'" If she wanted a divorce, she needn't go to such lengths—he would not refuse her. "I should think we had skill enough to adjust the terms of a separation without the wretchedness to all our family," Chamberlain wrote, "which these low people to whom it would seem that you confide your grievances & plans, will certainly bring about." Though he was angry, before closing the letter Chamberlain attempted to explain the personal impact of Fanny's actions. Her allegations and bitterness, he wrote, were "a very great trial ... more than all things put together—wounds, pains, toils, wrongs, & hatred of eager enemies."[40]

The exact role Chamberlain's wound played in his marital discord can't be known without definitive evidence. But his reference to the malady alongside other complicating elements indicates that he perceived a connection between the wound and his marriage troubles. The incident made Chamberlain's emasculation manifold: his genitals were painfully useless, his sexual relationship with his wife had changed, and Fanny was openly deriding him. Fanny had brought their deeply private relationship problems not only to their friends and neighbors in small Brunswick, but also, because Chamberlain was governor, to the people of Maine. Though his wound through the hips was common knowledge, the genital complications were not. "I am sorry to say this to you," Chamberlain told Fanny, "when I have so entirely confided in you & been so reassured of late in this confidence."[41] Was it possible that Fanny spoke to her untrustworthy friends about the most private parts of Chamberlain's life? The letter doesn't indicate what she revealed, but it does demonstrate Chamberlain's shaken confidence in her discretion.

The Chamberlains were hardly the only couple whose partnership changed due to the stresses and physical toll of the war. Lt. Col. Henry Boynton was shot in the groin while leading his men at Chickamauga. The ball cut through his spermatic cords, making it impossible for the young man to ever father children. When Boynton married in 1871, he and his wife were able to have a child by adopting Boynton's orphaned niece.[42] Genital wounds changed the terms of marriages. Col. Charles Johnson, after gunshot wounds to the legs and testicles, had to remind his wife that her hopes for another child were not to be: "Mary, that thing is 'played out'— or more properly and correctly or definitely speaking '*I* am played out'—I am sorry (for your sake) that I can not accomidate you."[43] We can't know what Charles and Mary's sexual relationship looked like—it may have been perfectly satisfying—but the injury altered any plans they might have had about growing their family. Indeed, Americans worried about the perception that disabled veterans were emasculated. Thus popular literature sometimes portrayed these men in ways that balanced disability with the ultimate proof of sexual ability—babies. An engraving entitled *The Empty Sleeve*, for example, features a soldier-amputee cradling a plump infant with one arm.[44]

Brian Craig Miller's recent work on Southern amputees suggests that wartime disability impacted relationships between men and women in negative and positive ways. Some women welcomed their soldiers home with open arms, prepared to face the challenges of disability together. But women also rejected incapacitated suitors, as did Sally Buchanan Preston, the sweetheart of luckless Confederate general and amputee John Bell Hood. Women disparaged disabled suitors as "wrecks." Fathers refused to bless their daughters' marriages to disabled soldiers for fear of their inability to provide for a family.[45] Even when women were open to their disabled beaus and husbands, Miller points out that "many of the veterans returned home physically or emotionally altered" by the war, making reintegration into the family difficult.[46] The Chamberlains narrowly avoided divorce by agreeing to live separately for the next several years. When Chamberlain returned home to Brunswick from the capital, he stayed with a neighbor, and Fanny often traveled. The couple reunited in the early 1870s, and though they remained affectionate until their deaths, they spent much of their time apart.[47]

Acute infections stemming from the vulnerably open fistula, often exacerbated by his dedication to work, punctuated Chamberlain's constant pain every few years.[48] By the spring of 1883, the general's health was worsening significantly. He had been postponing another surgery in hopes of keeping up with his demanding schedule, which involved traveling for speaking engagements and conducting his duties as president of Bowdoin. Chamberlain's physician, Joseph H. Warren of Boston, finally had to insist that he have the surgery immediately. Warren believed that the delay of treatment, exacerbated by Chamberlain's intense work schedule, had left his health in a precarious state. "The condition is now critical," Warren wrote. "You have worked too hard, & been neglected too long.... I shall not be responsible unless you obey these orders. Do not fail, do not hesitate, & do not linger."[49] The general had little choice but to resign his long-held post as president of Bowdoin College in the face of a long and arduous recovery away from Brunswick. Still, he strove to complete as much work as possible before taking his leave. After consulting with Dr. Warren, Chamberlain continued to lecture at Bowdoin until it was time to leave for his surgery. Even the *New York Times* noted his stubborn determination to keep working. "He has met the Senior Class regularly and sometimes twice a day," the paper reported in a note copied from Maine's *Portland Press*, "striving to complete as many lectures as possible before he should be obliged to give up."[50]

The surgery was performed on April 19, 1883, and initially appeared successful. As word circulated that Chamberlain had undergone an operation on his Petersburg wound, it became clear just how secretive the general had been about the effects of his disability. John Bigelow, former captain of the Ninth Massachusetts Battery, read of Chamberlain's situation in the newspaper and expressed surprise that the wound was still so troublesome. "From time to time when I have had the pleasure of meeting you," Bigelow wrote his friend, "you have spoken so lightly about your Petersburg wound, that I was led to believe it was not causing you trouble."[51] Even Fanny expressed shock at the seriousness of her husband's condition. She had not gone to Boston with Chamberlain, most likely because of her own poor health, and she wrote to him shortly after the surgery, declaring, "I'm afraid [I've had] ignorance of your illness for a long time."[52]

Chamberlain's procedure exposed his wound and its effects to the public. Journalists for Maine's *Portland Transcript* reported on the general's health in surprising detail and went on to detail the surgery. According to the paper's report, the general was under ether when Dr. Warren made "the necessary incisions and openings." From there, "portions of living flesh were taken in minute subdivisions from places near the opening where they could be spared, and delicately applied to the reconstruction of portions of the natural canal which had been taken away. A great number of stitches was rendered necessary."[53] If Chamberlain had hoped to conceal the extent and location of his injuries, the article spoiled that possibility. Although relatively vague in its descriptions of the wound's location, Maine readers of the *Transcript*'s account would have had little trouble gleaning what "canal" the newspaper referenced.

The *Transcript*'s detailing of Chamberlain's wound and reparative surgery bridged a gap between the public's fascination with veterans' visible traumas and ignorance of nonvisible ones. Northerners were fascinated with the bodies of disabled Union soldiers, which offered political and cultural reminders of the tragic but necessary sacrifices of the war years. Engravings and cartoons in popular magazines prominently featured amputees, as did poems, songs, and sentimental fiction. William Oland Bourne's left-handed penmanship contests placed amputees' writing in exhibits that able-bodied citizens could peruse and contemplate.[54] War wounds, visible and nonvisible, were considered simultaneously individual and communal. While a veteran's experience of a wound was personal, the nation considered such wounds collectively—the combined bloodletting of a nation.

Amputations were conspicuous reminders of the nation's wounds, but nonvisible wounds were often unavailable for public contemplation. Chamberlain's surgery, however, had given the *Transcript* the opportunity to consider less obvious wounds. The paper not only described Chamberlain's trauma in excruciating detail, but it also offered a lengthy contemplation on how modern medicine could repair such injuries. The surgery seemed to the *Transcript* to be an example of the miracles of modern medicine. "Man is not only wonderfully made, but is capable of being wonderfully mended," the article's author gushed. "Every particle of bone, every atom of skin or flesh is all alive and even ready to repair.... We may lose half our physical substance and be patched up again by the contributions of our friends." Physicians had the power to fix the human body completely, restoring it to proper working order with no lasting ill effects. "The human machine" could be taken apart and reassembled, then go on "ticking like an eight day clock."[55] According to the *Transcript*'s interpretation, Chamberlain's wound had been agonizing, but Dr. Warren had used medical ingenuity to fix it. In the public's mind, Dr. Warren's skillful surgery had healed Chamberlain and returned him to normality.

The *Transcript* reflected postwar Americans' hopes that veterans' horrific wounds might be easily mended, a hopefulness most commonly associated with the burgeoning prosthetics industry. In 1863, physician Oliver Wendell Holmes Sr. was filled with optimistic awe when he visited the Boston shop of famed prosthetics manufacturer B. Frank Palmer. The establishment hosted a group of soldier-amputees, whom Holmes dubbed unipeds, experimenting with their new legs. "At first they move with a good deal of awkwardness," Holmes observed, "but gradually the wooden limb seems to become, as it were, penetrated by the nerves, and the intelligence to run downwards until it reaches the last joint of the member." Holmes seemed to believe that these legs, though carved from wood, could be "penetrated by nerves" and become a living part of the body.[56]

To Holmes, Palmer's artificial legs offered a way to repair the "melancholy harvest" of limbs being reaped like so much wheat on the front lines. The physician delighted in demonstrations of the wooden leg. He asked a one-legged worker at the prosthetics shop to walk for him so that he might guess "which was Nature's leg and which Mr. Palmer's." The man walked the room until Holmes was sure "which was the leg of willow and which that of flesh and bone." He was amazed to learn that he had guessed the wrong leg: "No victim of the thimble-rigger's trickery was ever more completely taken in than we were by the contrivance of that ingenious Surgeon-Artist."[57] Palmer's wooden leg was virtually indistinguishable from the living one. It seemed possible that medical and technological ingenuity could make soldiers' bodies whole again, returning the wounded to the ranks of the productive and able-bodied and erasing the reminders of the horrors of the war.

It was possible for those amputees who used prosthetics to give the impression of wholeness, but that did not remove the image of the amputee from the public consciousness. When they were not being considered in terms of the wonders of prosthetic technology, amputees were portrayed in the popular media through sentimental works glorifying patriotic sacrifice. Sentimental stories and poetry featuring veterans who happily gave their limbs for the cause were commonplace in the postbellum decades.[58] One such poem, "The Veteran," appeared in *Harper's Weekly* in 1867. In this work, a former Union soldier, still wearing his worn-out uniform, leans on a crutch on a village green while telling tales from his army life in an attempt to sell medicinal salves. After selling some of his wares, the veteran pauses, and the narrator of the poem watches him closely:

> And while he paused in his simple strain
> Twas little he recked of trade or gain;
> For, lost in his tale, his soul had wrought
> A grander vision, a nobler thought.
> He thought of his country's triumph—the price
> Of his own most costly sacrifice;
> And a loving glance, suffused and dim,
> Fell down upon his shattered limb.
> I saw a tear on his eyelid flash—
> I saw it fall from the quivering lash;
> And he spake these words, unheard of men:
> "All that I gave I would give again!"

This veteran considers his lost leg intimately connected to the "grander vision." He even looks down "upon his shattered limb" lovingly, treasuring his offering given for "his country's triumph." Casting aside memories of the pain of the amputation or thoughts about the difficulties of a disabled life, the veteran murmurs that he would lose his limb again if asked.[59] A well-known song of the day, aptly named "The Empty Sleeve," is yet more pointed in identifying an amputation's symbolism:

> It tells of a battlefield of gore
> of the sabre's clash—of the cannon's roar. . . .
> It points to a time when that flag shall wave
> o'er a land where there breathes no cowering slave.[60]

Amputations, both real and imagined, reminded postwar Americans that veterans' sacrifices merited support, even as pension rolls swelled. More importantly, the removal of limbs came to represent the very meaning of the war. Chamberlain's wounds, though momentarily scrutinized in the *Portland Transcript*, became nonvisible again when Dr. Warren completed his procedure. After all, the newspaper ran a story implying that the general had been cured and his wound "restored." If Chamberlain wanted his own wounds to be part of the story of the war, he would have to reveal their scope and nature himself. No sentimental poetry would remind the public on his behalf that such hidden wounds deserved support—or, for that matter, that these wounds even continued to exist.

Chamberlain's experience was far from that of Holmes's unipeds or the old soldiers in mawkish stories. Dr. Warren might have been armed with the powers of modern medicine, but he was unable to "fix" the wound as the *Transcript* suggested. Rather than resolving Chamberlain's illness, the surgery brought a new kind of suffering. In July, the *New York Times* reported that the general's health was "not much improved," and that he would "never entirely recover from his wounds."[61] To compel himself to rest, Chamberlain moved to Domhegan, his summer home just outside of Brunswick, in hopes the sea air would prove healing. He wrote his sister that the surgeons were highly optimistic about his health after the surgery. But Chamberlain himself was skeptical. "The [wound] has been greatly helped, I *think*, by the operation & *may* be overcome," he wrote, adding, "The Doctor says I shall be better than for 20 years, but I take that at a discount, & rather hold my judgment in abeyance on that *point*."[62] His skepticism was prescient. The fistula that the surgery had attempted to close soon reopened, and Chamberlain's struggles with infection and illness began anew.

In 1892, Chamberlain applied for an increase in his pension. The return of the fistula meant increased infection, and the surgery had only exacerbated his chronic pain. Affidavits from army comrades, most notably former Union Fifth Corps major general Fitz John Porter, who asserted that Chamberlain was an "almost helpless invalid," supported the general's application for an increase.[63] There was little doubt that Chamberlain needed the money. Thanks to his wartime officership, his pension allotments were higher than an average payout. But they still were not enough to cover his medical costs and provide for his family. Fanny was gradually going blind and required near constant care, and the Chamberlains' son Wyllys, never successful in finding a career, still relied on his father for financial support. The family's finances had been tight since Chamberlain had left Bowdoin for the surgery in 1883. Once he had recovered enough from the surgery to work again, Chamberlain had tried his hand at various new ventures—real estate investor, art school president, railroad executive—but he succeeded at none.

Pension Bureau officials denied the requested increase, insisting they needed more proof that the wound directly caused the "alleged" infections.

More importantly, they would need some proof that Chamberlain was, as Fitz John Porter had indicated, truly helpless. In other words, the general would need another medical examination. Thomas Ingram, medical referee of the Pension Bureau, wrote a note explaining what information the bureau needed: "Can he dress, undress, eat, and walk without assistance? For which of the requirements of life does he need the aid of another? What disability confines him to the house or bed and is it permanent in its present degree? Make the examination through giving reasons for all opinions expressed."[64] Clearly, Chamberlain would have to demonstrate utter reliance on others for survival in order to get the much-needed pension increase. He faced the trap disability scholar Tobin Siebers calls "compulsory able-bodiedness." As Siebers notes, while individuals are expected to act and appear as nondisabled as possible, they must disclose their disabilities in order to access support. In turn, their disclosures make them vulnerable to greater discrimination.[65] Chamberlain undeniably needed help when he was acutely ill, but he was able to move and work independently between attacks. In the years after Petersburg, Chamberlain had learned how to work with his body through its pain and illness, crafting an image of able-bodiedness. In order to receive the pension increase, he would now need to display his private wounds and swear that he was entirely disabled—that he was a dependent, unable to overcome war trauma.

Chamberlain scheduled an additional medical examination but got another severe infection while awaiting it. When the infection didn't improve, he traveled to New York City, where the family was living part of the time, for medical treatment. There, he was far from the board of examinations the Pension Bureau had asked him to see in Maine. "Since coming to New York," he explained to the bureau, "I have been very much disabled, and on the 29th of December last the inflammation culminated in a severe acute attack, which has kept me in a condition of complete disability and great suffering ever since."[66] This "attack of inflammation of the wounded parts," as Chamberlain described it, had already lasted seven months. He would not be able to travel back to Maine for the examination. When Chamberlain eventually arranged to be examined in New York, the surgeon agreed that his pain and sickness were severe. Yet the surgeon also testified to the Pension Bureau that since the general's acute infections were only episodic, he was not completely dependent on others. Moreover, Chamberlain's muscular build was good, and, though his hair was getting white, he showed no evidence of "general debility."[67] As Chamberlain was not dependent enough, the increase was denied again. His brother Tom, acting as his pension attorney, appealed the decision, and the bureau ordered yet another examination. This time, Chamberlain refused it. A September 1893 note scrawled in his pension file states, "Atty. Chamberlain inf'd that as client declines to comply with this exam no further action can be taken."[68] It seems that the general had had enough of putting himself on display for the Pension Bureau.

Chamberlain was far from alone in his experience with the Pension Bureau. As the bureau's rolls swelled in the final decades of the nineteenth century, the public grew increasingly frustrated with federal spending on veterans. Decades had passed since the close of the Civil War, and the feelings of indebtedness toward disabled Union veterans had waned. While this sense of responsibility diminished, postwar Americans also became increasingly skeptical of veterans' disabilities. Harvard University president Charles Eliot, a harsh critic of the pension system, voiced this distrust: "One cannot tell whether a pensioner of the United States is a disabled soldier or sailor or a perjured pauper who has foisted himself upon the public treasury."[69] Amputees, whose wounds were fairly easily confirmed, were mostly exempt from suspicion. In the minds of average Americans accustomed to seeing amputees in the pages of popular magazines, amputation spoke clearly of the sacrifices of the war years. The wartime loss of a limb was difficult, though not impossible, to fake. Instead, increased scrutiny shifted to those who bore nonvisible disabilities. These ailments were numerous and diverse, harder to categorize, and harder—sometimes nearly impossible—to confirm. How did one adequately prove that a back problem truly originated in a war injury, or that chronic diarrhea stemmed from disease contracted in camp? Increasingly, veterans with these less visible and more nebulous disabilities encountered obstacles in the pension system.[70]

Other veterans with nonvisible wounds chose to make their injuries more visible in order to increase their pension payments. Henry A. Barnum of the 127th New York was shot through the front left of his hip bone at the Battle of Malvern Hill in 1862. As with Chamberlain's wound, the ball passed through Barnum's body, and surgeons considered the trauma fatal. After a fairly dramatic, and no doubt painful, experience in which he was taken prisoner while in the field hospital and transported dozens of miles to be exchanged, Barnum was eventually transferred to his home in Syracuse, New York. Unsurprisingly, during the weeks-long journey from Libby Prison to his home, infection had set in. In order to save Barnum's life, a physician cleaned the wound of bone fragments and instructed him to wear a tent, a kind of soft fabric plug that would keep the wound open and draining. Over the course of two years, during which Barnum was given command of the 149th New York and promoted to brigadier general, the wound developed two abscesses. To prevent further infections, Dr. Lewis D. Sayre strung an oakum seton, effectively a rope, through the wound to encourage it to drain. The oakum was eventually replaced by long pieces of candlewick, which Barnum wore, threaded through the open wound, for the remainder of his life.[71]

Unlike Chamberlain's wound, however, Barnum's became famous. Dr. George Otis, curator of the Army Medical Museum, which the Surgeon General's Office established during the war, requested that Major Barnum's wound be photographed for inclusion in *The Medical and Surgical History of the War of the Rebellion*. Barnum was photographed at the museum in Washington, DC, in 1865. The image was subsequently displayed in the museum and published in *The Medical and Surgical History*.[72] Barnum used the picture to lend credibility to his original pension application in 1866, but this was not the only photograph made of the wound. The pension file references this image yet includes an additional one, featuring a considerably older Barnum in military uniform. He signed the photograph, scrawling his signature beneath the line of what appears to be either a rope or rod passing through his open wound. The image was made sometime in the early 1880s, but there is no indication whether it was made by or for the Army Medical Museum.[73]

When Barnum sought a pension increase in 1888, he wrote to George Lockwood of the Pension Bureau, explaining that his distress was increasing: "My sufferings in the past year have been much greater than formerly on account of frequent & severe abscesses caused by exfoliated dead bone." He stated that he would include a photograph of the wound, then remembered that a copy of the 1880 photograph was already in his files. Barnum told Lockwood, "If you do not find such a one in my papers, let me know and I will send one for inspection & *return* as I have no other."[74] Maintaining a visual record of his wound must have been important to Barnum. More photographs in which a young Barnum displays the wound while in civilian clothing appear to have been taken privately soon after the war.[75]

It was not just photographs that documented the injury. In 1881, when Pres. James Garfield lay suffering from a gunshot wound in Washington, DC, Barnum apparently was summoned to the capital so that the president's surgeons could compare their patient's open wound to his own. The *Syracuse Courier* reported in the summer of 1881, "General H. A. Barnum, who for nineteen years has carried an open bullet wound through the body . . . and is now wearing a rubber draining tube through the track of the ball, passing through the left ilium, was this morning telegraphed to go to Washington for personal examination by the President's surgeons, with a view of such

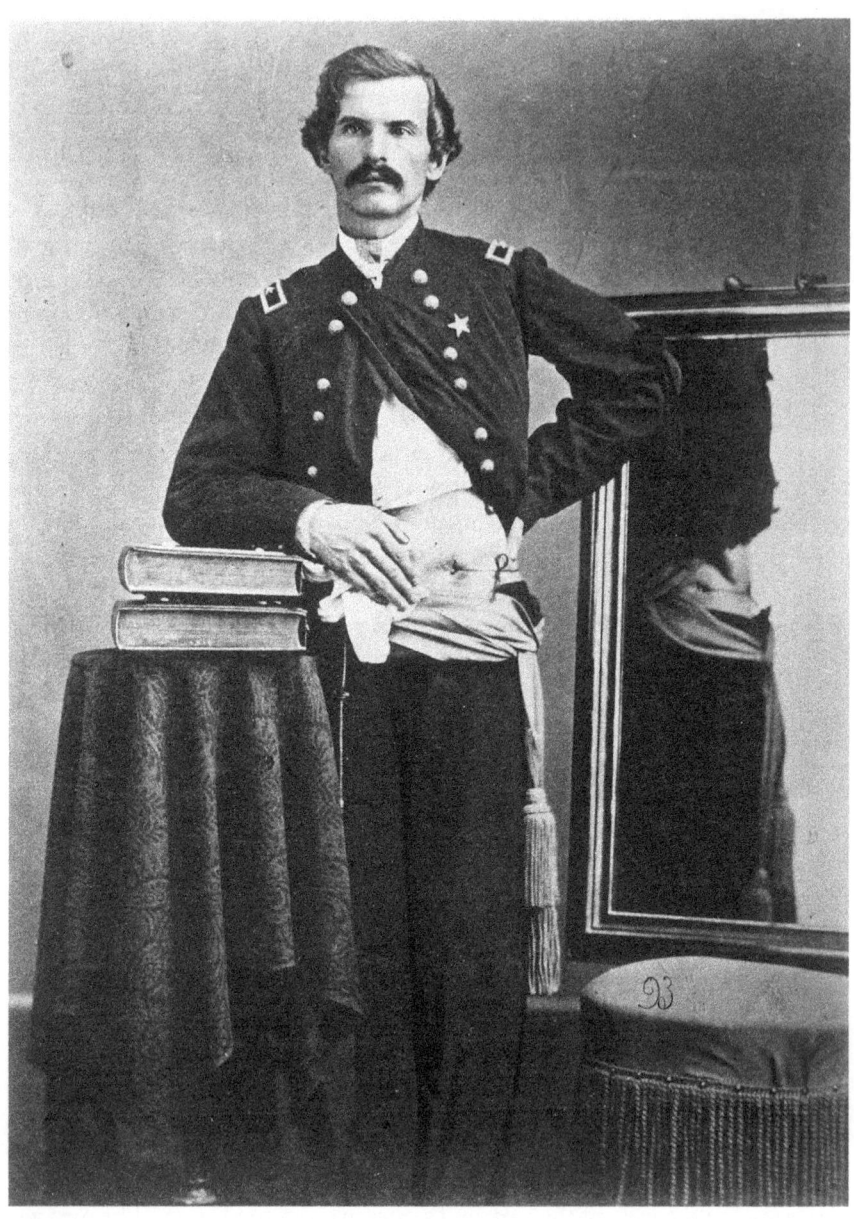

FIGURE 7. Henry Barnum. *Recovery after a Penetrating Gunshot Wound of the Abdomen, with Perforation of the Left Ilium* (SP 93). OHA 82 Surgical Photographs Collection, Otis Historical Archives, National Museum of Health and Medicine, Silver Spring, MD.

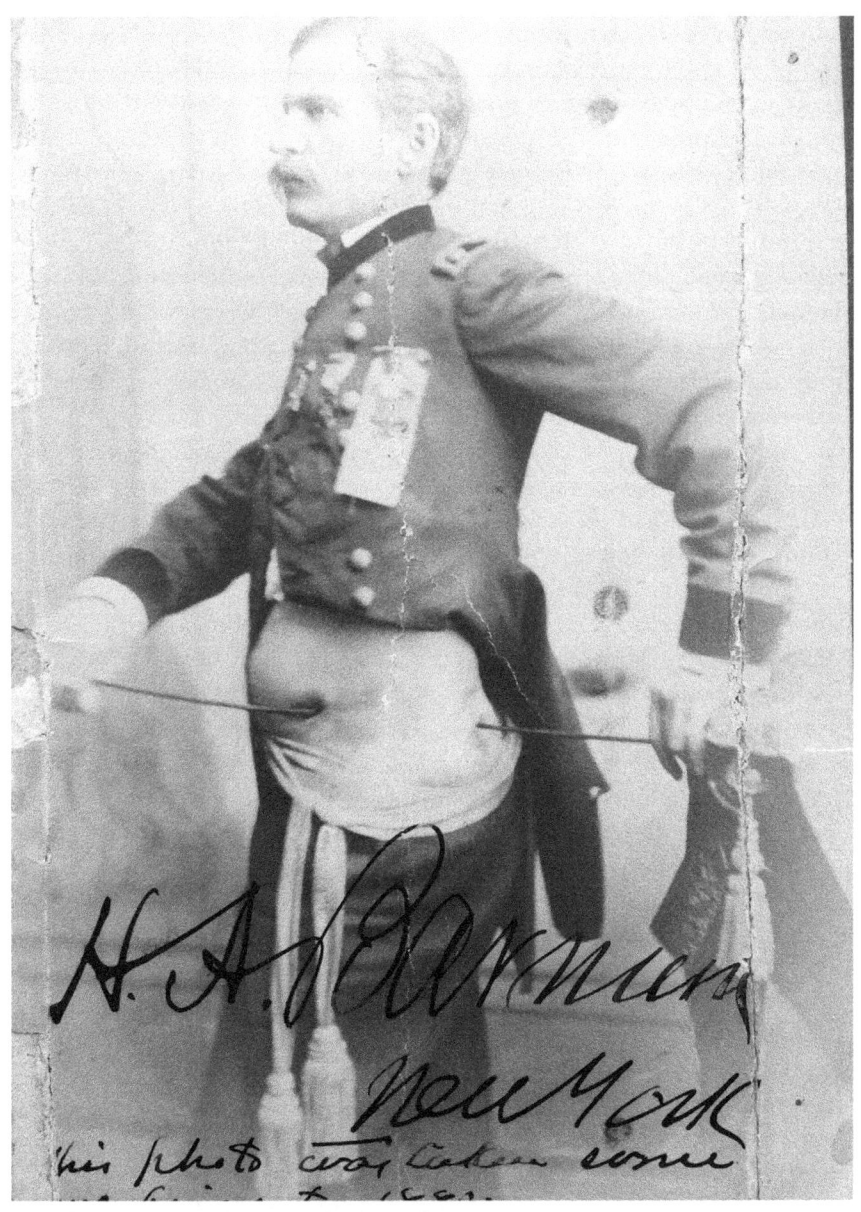

FIGURE 8. Henry Barnum, ca. 1881. Henry A. Barnum Military Pension Records, certificate 78,753, National Archives and Records Administration, Washington, DC.

information as his care may give with reference to the President's wound."⁷⁶ Not only was Barnum's wound publicized, it was continuing to do a service to the nation by offering its painful lessons to the surgeons attending the assassinated president.

Public awareness of Barnum's wounds seemed to pay off. In August 1889, when Barnum was awarded the Medal of Honor, former New York governor Alonzo Cornell held a reception in his honor. The invitations included some bitter criticisms of the federal government's neglect of its veterans. Barnum was a "patriotic officer," Cornell wrote, who "for more than twenty-five years [had] borne with uncomplaining fortitude painful wounds received on the field of battle as well as the seeming neglect of the Government in the appropriate recognition of his extraordinary services."⁷⁷ The following year, a special act of Congress raised Barnum's pension to one hundred dollars.

Chamberlain had no such luck. Though he, too, received the Medal of Honor in 1893, by the turn of the century, the general's financial situation was growing tenuous.⁷⁸ Friends and old comrades undertook a letter campaign asking that he be given a patronage position in the port of Portland, Maine. President McKinley agreed that Chamberlain deserved a patronage post but gave him the job of port surveyor. The position was less prestigious than the one he had hoped for, but Chamberlain nonetheless kept it until his death.⁷⁹ His health grew increasingly worse with age, but he never stopped pushing himself. In the final years before his death, the old veteran worked at the port, wrote and published essays about the war, and helped to plan the fiftieth anniversary reunion at Gettysburg in 1913, though he was too ill to attend. In the winter of 1914, a final infection of Chamberlain's war wounds lead to pneumonia. Even at eighty-five, he sought to defeat his old enemy. "I am passing through dark waters!" he wrote in a dictated letter to his sister. "The Dr. thinks I will land once more on this shore. I seem to be gaining deliverance from the particular disease which caused me unspeakable agony and gaining strength from the condition to which it reduced me."⁸⁰ This time, however, there was no amount of work Chamberlain could do to fight the wound. A month later, he was dead.

Joshua Lawrence Chamberlain spent most of his years with a disability that significantly changed his life, yet few would categorize him as disabled. His passing was possible because he exercised what power he had to adhere to standards of able-bodied manhood, but also because his life confounded assumptions about disabled people. Chamberlain blurred the lines of what it meant to be a disabled war hero in the Civil War era. His portraits depict no

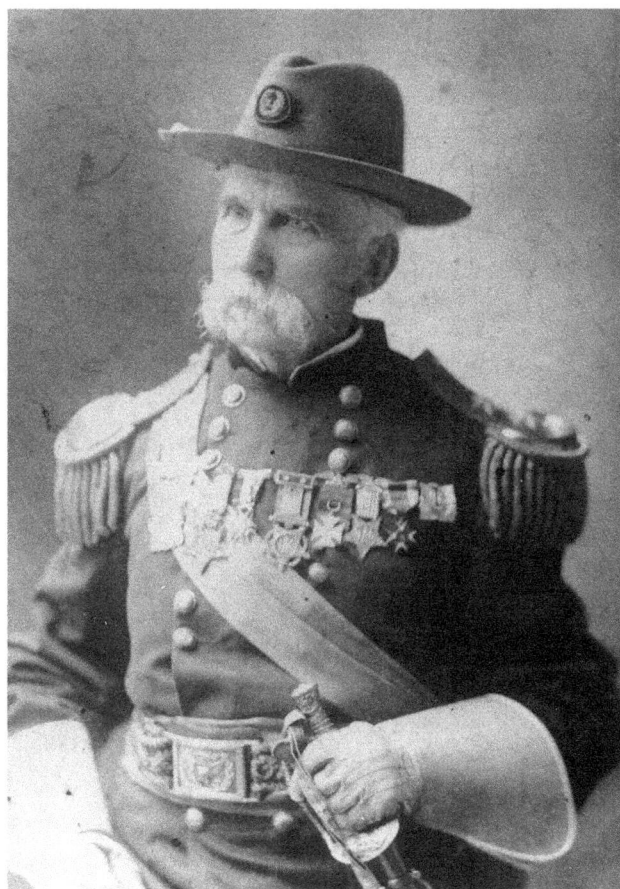

FIGURE 9. Joshua Lawrence Chamberlain in full uniform, undated. Local Call Number M27, Bowdoin College Archives, Brunswick, ME.

visible wounds. He didn't contemplate his infirmities in his public writings. He was successful and satisfied in his later life. Nonetheless, Chamberlain grappled with chronic pain and sickness, struggled with the Pension Bureau, and was subject to the surgeon's scalpel and the media's scrutiny. The most intimate parts of his body and his life were drastically altered. His public postwar writing is proof that he considered the war important, and that he understood on an abstract level that bodily sacrifice was critical to the Union victory. But the general took a darker tone in private writings when considering the role his own wounds may have played. As a case study, Chamberlain calls for a more nuanced interpretation of Civil War disability, one that makes space for a diversity of experience and allows soldiers and veterans to feel contradictory emotions.

Chamberlain seemed in so many ways to be the ideal Union soldier. This persona might have sealed his place in the pantheon of Civil War leaders, but it also worked against him when it came to pension support. He was never submissive enough, helpless enough, disabled enough. The full paradox of the pension experience, however, is that men who declared helplessness in their requests for support were not rewarded as one might expect. Rather, as in Chamberlain's experience, they were met with suspicion and scorn.

CHAPTER 5

Man or Mercenary

On February 4, 1887, Pres. Grover Cleveland vetoed seven bills—rejecting more legislation in a day than many of his predecessors had in their entire term of office.[1] All seven were private pension bills, acts of Congress to provide governmental support to Civil War veterans and their family members whom the Pension Bureau did not support. One of the vetoed measures was for Abraham P. Griggs, veteran of the First New Jersey Cavalry. Griggs had received a disability discharge for "debility" in 1863, but the Pension Bureau had repeatedly rejected his requests for support. No doubt frustrated, Griggs had sought recourse through his congressman, joining hundreds of other veterans and dependents who sought private legislation to secure pensions in the late nineteenth century.

After carefully perusing Griggs's pension file, which included statements from the old soldier's discharging surgeons, Cleveland was unmoved. Though the cavalryman had been hospitalized for rheumatism for nearly a year in 1863, his physicians had written in his discharge, "We do not believe him sick, or that he has been sick, but completely worthless. He is obese and a malingerer to such an extent that he is almost an imbecile—worthlessness, obesity, and imbecility and laziness."[2] So degraded was Griggs's character that the surgeons deemed him unqualified even for the Invalid Corps. Cleveland vetoed the bill, stating his belief that, based on the opinion of Griggs's doctors, the Pension Bureau was justified in its rejection. But something about Griggs's case impelled Cleveland to detail the problems with the man's pension file in a letter to Congress explaining the veto. In addition to citing the surgeons' harsh words about Griggs, Cleveland repeated the findings of the veteran's most recent medical examination. Surgeons had found no overt signs of disability despite the man's complaints of heart trouble, rheumatism, and sunstroke. Convinced of Griggs's able-bodiedness, his examiners had added, "His hands are hard indicating an ability to work."[3] Regardless of what lingering effects of war Abraham Griggs carried, his able hands betrayed him.

For the first fifteen years following the surrender at Appomattox, the Republican and Democratic Parties supported the pension system, each hoping to capitalize on the massive veteran vote. Northerners awash in gratitude for the victors of the Union overwhelmingly supported the system established under the 1862 Act to Grant Pensions. While there were some complaints about fraud in the system, a plateau in pension applications a decade after the war placated critics who believed the payouts had reached their height. The 1879 Arrears Act, which guaranteed veterans a lump-sum pension payment dating back to the origin of their disability, led to a significant increase in the number of pensioned veterans.[4] The Arrears Act received bipartisan support, as both parties courted the veteran vote, but the harmony was not to last. Debates erupted in the 1880s over the existence and proper spending of a federal surplus. Democrats hoped to lower taxes and tariffs; Republicans saw the surplus as a way to woo veteran voters by supporting generous pensions.[5] The perception that veterans were lining their pockets with large pensions at the expense of the American taxpayer, coupled with annoyance at the greedy behavior of the Grand Army of the Republic and other lobbyists, made the last decades of the century a particularly contentious period. Soldiers' bodies were at the center of the debate.

Decades earlier, at the war's end, the civilian public could not express its gratitude to Union soldiers more emphatically. As Brian Jordan notes, there could hardly have been a stronger statement than the banner that hung from the Treasury Building in May 1865 proclaiming, "The Only National Debt We Can Never Repay Is The Debt We Owe Our Victorious Union Soldiers."[6] The state did endeavor to repay the debt—pension law slowly grew more inclusive until nearly all veterans had benefits by 1915.[7] But as Democratic concern about government spending turned the swelling pension rolls into a political football, a suspicious public more closely scrutinized the ranks of veterans in an attempt to separate the deserving from the undeserving. While few Americans were ready to back away from pensions for the *true* victors of the Union, many critics were more than happy to see the undeserving cut off. Weeding out these individuals meant critically analyzing veterans—supposedly the best men the country had to offer—to determine which among them were pretenders. The result was a renewed debate over what constituted a legitimate disability, and also over which soldiers had the privilege of claiming such a disability. Debates played out in the pages of the partisan press were translated into action as the state, whether in the form of a pension clerk or the president himself, rewarded soldiers who fit its notions of manhood and disability, and rejected those who did not.

In 1894, Union veteran John Dodge was reportedly granted a sizable pension for partial paralysis. Shortly after this award, he applied for an increase of his payments, this time claiming that he was also blind. Suspicious, the Pension Bureau assigned Dodge's case to a special examiner, a bureaucrat charged with the most difficult and perplexing pension cases. Intent on proving to the examiner that he was, indeed, disabled, Dodge visited the Pension Bureau in person, "dragging himself along on crutches and wearing blue googles."[8] The bureau official still was not entirely convinced. Another examiner followed Dodge to his home, where he watched the veteran cast his crutches and goggles aside and move around with ease. Dodge's pension was revoked, and a warrant was issued for his arrest, but he escaped before he could be apprehended.[9]

As James Marten points out, the Gilded Age press was a major driver of the pension debates, and the era's journalists were obsessed with pension fraud, especially cases as blatant as Dodge's.[10] The belief that fraudulent claims bloated the Civil War pension system was pervasive but false. Investigations to weed out unauthorized pensions, launched in 1873, 1876, and 1879, resulted in the dropping of only 0.5 percent of the total pensions. Another investigation in 1893 claimed to have found hundreds of bad claims, but, as Theda Skocpol concludes, "even if we suppose ... that 'hundreds' of fraudulent cases revealed by the 1893 investigations led to as many as 900 dropped cases, that would still be fewer than one-tenth of one percent of all the pensions on the rolls in that year."[11] There were certainly people who conned the Pension Bureau, but the system was far from riddled with fraud. Rather, breathless media accounts of unworthy veterans fed the perception of widespread corruption. The notion that an undeserving population was living off the United States Treasury played into Americans' well-established tendency to see conspiracy everywhere.[12]

Conspiracy certainly seemed possible when stories of fraudulent cases appeared regularly in newspapers and magazines. Missouri's *Jackson Citizen*, for instance, reported on the case of John Stockwell, who stole the papers of a deceased veteran and applied for the man's pension in his place. Also in Missouri, the *Kansas City Times* printed the story of James V. Busby, who did the same.[13] In some cases, it wasn't fraud as much as it was audacity on the part of soldiers with appalling military records. North Dakota's *Grand Forks Daily Herald* printed a portion of a letter that one particularly bold, impatient veteran wrote to his congressman. The "would-be pensioner" explained that he had enlisted and taken a furlough of his own accord when his request for leave had been denied. The man had then enlisted in a new regiment, served for a few months, and taken another unauthorized furlough. "Before I could enlist again the war was over," he wrote. "I don't think the government could be mean enough to beat me out of my bounty and pension on that account."[14] Stories such as these represented only a tiny fraction of the claims the Pension Bureau processed. However, they occupied a large space in the popular imagination and fed the belief that the ranks of the aging Union army were not so heroic as some might believe.

It was soldiers with bad records who seemed the most infuriating in their boldness. The Rockford, Illinois, *Daily Register* published an article stating, "Those whose career in the service was indeed dishonorable, the bounty-jumpers, deserters, and malingerers, all the gangs who entered the government service for other than patriotic ends and by unsoldierly conduct justified their comrades in sending them out of it with dishonor, should be kept off the pension roll."[15] This article reflected a tendency to categorize unworthy soldiers into three groups: "mercenaries" and "bounty-jumpers," who sought to gain from their military service; "deserters," who were dishonorably discharged or otherwise failed to serve nobly; and "malingerers," who faked or exaggerated wounds and illnesses for gain. Each category stood in opposition to the "true soldier of Union," a volunteer who gave his body to the cause without regard to risk or reward, who suffered his wounds quietly, and who, like Cincinnatus, returned to the farm after the war. According to this idealized trope, true soldiers would never beg the government for support or advocate for liberalized pension legislation. Rather, they advocated *less* support in order to protect the legacy of the vaunted Union army.

The mercenary fighting for a paycheck rather than out of a sense of duty was anathema to the citizen-soldier ethos of the Union army. Even during the war, soldiers motivated by money were considered inferior. As previously discussed, Roberts Bartholow believed that men who received bounties to enlist were more prone to malingering.[16] Mercenaries fought because they relished war for war's sake or received financial incentive. The citizen-soldier took up arms only out of a sense of manful duty and happily set them down again at war's end. Similarly, soldiers and civilians looked down on conscripts, who hadn't even made a conscious decision to enlist. Those who waited for bribes or were forced to fight for their country were poor men indeed—or perhaps, as one soldier commented, men who were motivated by money were "no men at all."[17]

The true soldier of the Union, the critical Gilded Age press insisted, was the citizen-soldier. A writer for the *New York Herald* protested pension spending by declaring that Union soldiers had volunteered without hope of compensation: "What we are proudest of is that they were not hirelings. No thought of hard cash prompted them to duty. The motives that urged them were of the most unselfish and holy character."[18] Of course, this argument required a bit of creative remembering. All Union soldiers received pay for their services and were generally pretty thrilled when the paymaster visited camp.[19] Other critics believed that the bounty system, which encouraged enlistment with significant sums of money, made some veterans mercenaries and others citizen-soldiers. Harvey W. Scott, editor of the *Portland Oregonian*, put the distinction succinctly: "Of the Northern armies more than a million men received large bounties to induce them to enter the service. These men were certainly not heroes, and probably never thought of themselves as anything but men under obligation to take certain risks for a certain amount of money."[20] Reigniting a talking point about a subset of soldiers from decades prior was more than an odd tactic—it was a dog whistle. Veterans who lobbied for increased benefits and more generous pension legislation were the moral equivalent of a peacetime mercenary.

The accusation that the ranks of Union veterans contained such immoral men intensified in the late 1880s, when Republicans in Congress, urged by the Grand Army of the Republic, proposed the Dependent Pension Bill. Grover Cleveland quickly vetoed this new legislation, which would offer a pension to all disabled veterans, whether or not war service had caused their disability. The bill had nevertheless raised pension critics' ire. According to Mark Summers, the 1880s saw an increase in political nostalgia for the war as Republicans focused more than ever on Union victors' courage to justify broadening pension benefits.[21] In response, frustrated critics drew a sharper line between good and bad soldiers in an attempt to criticize the bloated pension system without alienating true heroes.

The specter of yet a more inclusive pension bill drew additional declarations that true Union veterans would reject payment for their service. Even if so-called mercenaries were wounded in the line of duty, critics claimed, they deserved no recompense. The *St. Louis Republic* drew a distinction between different kinds of disabled veterans: "The volunteer and the mercenary should not be left on the same level. The hireling, disabled in service, is entitled to no gratitude from the government."[22] Any changes to the laws, the editors wrote, should offer extra support for the "patriotic volunteer." These funds should be disbursed only when a veteran was too elderly to work, which would "put his name on a roll of honor" separate from mercenaries. To do otherwise would elevate the "impudent and rapacious" mercenaries—those most stridently demanding pensions—rather than the true volunteers. Though it might have seemed that a "red badge of courage" was all a soldier needed to prove his manhood, a wound would not make up for failure to selflessly answer the call of duty.

However, it wasn't realistic to expect that all citizen-soldiers would refuse all postwar remuneration. Nearly everyone agreed that at least some Union veterans deserved aid, and thousands of soldiers were already pensioned.[23] In a perfect world, however, men would serve without any expectation of government support in exchange. For some, the idea didn't seem that far-fetched. One only needed to look south to find soldiers demonstrating superior manhood by surviving without support. It seemed to some that Confederate veterans, who were ineligible for federal pensions, were (by necessity) more self-reliant than their pampered Union counterparts. In its continuous pushing for more legislation, *Portland Oregonian* editorialist Harvey Scott wrote, "the Republican party will succeed in making the Confederate soldier the only hero of the war."[24] The South's approach to supporting its veterans was more manly than that of the North: "The South does take better care of its officers than the North, but it does it man fashion through politics and not through pension acts."[25] In another article, Scott praised Confederate veterans' "manly example" of handling difficulty with acceptance and fortitude.[26]

The *New York Herald* was even more pointed in exalting the superior manhood of Confederate veterans: "They threw all their energies, all their zeal, into the work first for self-support, and next for the upbuilding of their section. No pensions for them; no back pay; no army of claim agents to assist them to a permanent condition of respectable beggary. Even the maimed and those whose bodies were wasted by disease entered the struggle for existence without the least expectation of assistance from any quarter, and as a result we see a work accomplished more marvellous, more honorable, more enduring than any of their achievements on the field."[27] Thus the Confederacy's soldiers, not the Union's, embodied the citizen-soldier ethos. While the absence of monetary support had raised Confederate veterans to manful honor in the postwar years, pensions had degraded Union veterans into grasping mendicants and mercenaries.

But this description of Confederate moral superiority was a rosy oversimplification. Initially, most disabled former Rebels did go without government assistance. They relied on assistance from individual states, which were too economically strapped to offer much beyond a small stipend or access to prosthetics. But rather than living a "marvellous" life, many disabled Confederate veterans relied on private charity or lived in poverty—the very scenario the federal pension system had been created to avoid. Several former Confederate states eventually offered pensions late in the century. These benefits used the same quarterly payments and a similar degree-rating system as the federal government, but payments were low.[28]

Former Confederate states' debates over pensions reflected the same gendered fear as federal debates: that paying old soldiers undermined the spirit of "true" soldiers, who fought purely out of devotion to the southland. In Arkansas, legislators bitterly argued a proposed 1891 Pension Act, with one lawmaker asserting, "Patriots do not go out and fight to be rewarded with pensions and bounties."[29] As Brian Craig Miller argues, many politicians believed that "if a southern veteran, no matter his physical condition, asked for a pension, he diminished his masculine stature among his peers."[30] How to best support ailing veterans without challenging their manhood was a necessary and contentious question in the North and in the South. Some critics of the federal system might have considered the southern situation more masculinizing, but the reality was that disabled former Confederates faced significant poverty, dependency, and degradation because of the lack of adequate state support.[31]

The second category critics lumped bad veterans into was that of deserter. Desertion carried such a heavy stigma into the postwar period that five states—Kansas, Pennsylvania, Wisconsin, New York, and Vermont—disenfranchised those who had been dishonorably discharged from the Union army.[32] In some cases, the categories of mercenary and deserter overlapped. Bounty jumpers, men who enlisted to receive a bounty, then deserted and reenlisted in another unit to draw a second bounty, were both soldiers for hire and deserters. Another concern was men who might not have left the service permanently but skulked, shirked, or straggled. Former brigadier general Francis Barlow, complaining of the numbers of dishonorable shirkers receiving pensions, recalled the skulkers he saw at the Battle of Antietam, when he had been taken, wounded, from the front line: "I was amazed to see the number of stragglers who were amusing themselves in the rear of the troops who were fighting in the front. The country in the rear was filled with soldiers broken up and scattered from their comrades, who were having 'picnics.' They were lying under trees, sleeping, cooking their coffee or other rations, and amusing themselves outside of the enemy's fire." These cowardly men, he complained, still applied for pensions.

Clear cases of deserters applying for pensions appalled critics and further proved the argument against expanding pension access. "Nobody is surprised now at the sort of people to whom are given pensions, because the service is carried on as a party electioneering business," railed the editors of the New Orleans *Times-Picayune*. The case of Russell Cole, formerly of the First New York Cavalry, particularly infuriated the journalists. Cole, it seemed, had been captured and had for some reason told his Confederate captors that he wished to fight for them. Decades later, Cole applied for a pension based on a disability incurred in the service. His application was initially rejected but approved eventually, and he was granted a pension. Cole refuted claims that he was a deserter by explaining that he had only joined the Confederates to avoid dying slowly in one of their notorious prison camps and increase his chances of escape. This justification failed to impress the *Picayune*: "Under [Benjamin Harrison's] administration, a deserter, it appears, is as good as the truest and bravest veteran that ever stood to the flag through four years of storm and battle."[33]

The third, and perhaps the most shameful, class of bad veterans was the malingerer. Malingering violated moral codes of manhood, undermined unit cohesion, and thus carried steep repercussions during the war. As mentioned in chapter 2, the charge was often made against soldiers who used poor health to excuse dereliction of duty or straggling. Similarly, accusations of malingering lodged against veterans were often used to undermine the legitimacy of their applications to the Pension Bureau. For critics of the expanding pension system, malingering became something of a catchall charge against any men who failed to live up to the masculine and heroic expectations for veterans.

Malingerers were deceivers and cowards, but they were also men who sought support they didn't merit. Many critics believed that, just as cowardly soldiers attempted to feign illness to avoid a hard march or engagement, some pension seekers invented or exaggerated ailments to get cash from the government. "In other words," stated an editorial in the *New York Sun*, "the malingerer who was busy in 1863 or 1864 deceiving the army surgeons in order to escape the hardships of duty or to avoid the dangers of battle, has as his counterpart in the malingerer of 1897 who feigns or exaggerates trifling bodily ailments in order to get a pension."[34] Malingering actually called the worthiness of all veterans into question. The *Sun* noted that it was a commonly held fallacy that "because so many of the Union soldiers were patriotic, self-sacrificing, devoted heroes, incapable of defrauding the Government which they loved and defended, all or nearly all of the veterans are such." The *Sun* then issued a crucial warning: "A man may be an old soldier and at the same time a malingerer, a fraud, and a swindler."³⁵ It was not enough to have served; an old soldier's worth hinged on his record and his manhood.

Tense public debate over the worth of certain veterans created a fraught situation for disabled former Union soldiers. As pressure mounted to combat fraud and root out bad soldiers, the vagaries of the pension application process became more pronounced. The Pension Bureau had never accepted applications wholesale. An estimated 28 percent of applications were rejected between 1862 and 1875, but as the century wore on, the bureau placed increased scrutiny on claims.³⁶ Influenced by concerns about veterans' worthiness, the application system allowed the Pension Bureau to "sift out the wheat from this army chaff."³⁷ In order to perform this sifting, examiners scrutinized applications for proof of mercenaries, deserters, and malingerers, while also seeking evidence of true soldiers of Union. Veterans, therefore, strove to fit themselves into this idealized image. A pattern emerged in successful applications: the veteran had been healthy and able-bodied on enlistment, and had served dutifully through the war before being tragically cut down with a disability that kept him from supporting himself or his family. Critical to the successful applicant's tale were the details that the soldier had worked diligently while able-bodied, and that he *wanted* to continue working but was limited by his wounded or diseased body.

This process was a delicate negotiation, but one that was integral to proving a veteran's worth. "That balancing act was especially necessary," historian Jalynn Olsen Padilla suggests, "as . . . American men became increasingly interested in their physical appearance and athletic ability." Pension applications' emphasis on the male body reflected a shift in manhood and labor in post–Civil War America. In the antebellum decades, middle-class manhood had emphasized self-control, gentility, and morality. Physicality had been associated with the working class.³⁸ The intense bodily exertion of the war years, coupled with anxieties over the state of American masculinity in the Gilded Age, placed a greater focus on the male body. The belief that American men needed to live a more "strenuous life," to borrow Theodore Roosevelt's phrase, was driven by concerns about the state of the white race as well as concerns over nervous diseases, such as neurasthenia, that plagued genteel white men.³⁹ In an effort to prove their manhood and stem the effects of the "overcivilization" of the marketplace, Gilded Age men were encouraged to develop physical prowess through weight lifting, hunting, and sports. Even clothing drew more attention to the male form, as changes in men's fashions emphasized muscular limbs and barrel chests.⁴⁰ In this atmosphere, veterans found themselves working to prove that they *had* been ideal men before the war and that they could no longer meet this standard. This balancing act meant that the class of men that had once been held up as the epitome of American masculinity had little choice but to accentuate their weakness and neediness in order to win support.

Yet even the most artfully crafted narrative could not withstand the Pension Bureau's exacting notions of disability. As chapter 1 indicates, the Invalid Corps tied its definitions of disability to a soldier's productivity. Likewise, pension legislation defined disability strictly by the degree to which a veteran was able to earn a living by manual labor.⁴¹ During the 1860s, that designation seemed straightforward; the majority of enlisted men in the Union army worked in a profession that required some degree of physical labor. As more men transitioned from blue-collar to white-collar work in the post–Civil War era, however, the definition of a veteran's disability remained tied to a form of work many of them did not perform.⁴² More importantly, linking a former soldier's pensionable worth to his capacity for manual labor meant compensating his potential productivity instead of his medical expenses, pain, or required accommodations. Some savvy veterans managed to work around this new stipulation. Successful pension attorney Edgar North supplied affidavits declaring his inability to perform manual labor—though he had never earned a living in that manner and continued to work as an attorney.⁴³ Most, however, were not so lucky. Instead, they faced suspicion when they offset small pension payouts by continuing to run their farms or businesses, only to have their apparent ability to work used against them.

Certain disabilities were deemed obviously incompatible with manual labor. Amputations had clear implications for a soldier's ability to pursue a manual trade.⁴⁴ Other conditions seemed similarly straightforward. Cyrus Davis, for instance, had been a farm laborer at the time of his enlistment, but became almost entirely blind after he was shot in the face at the Battle of Smithfield Crossing in 1864. Upon reviewing Davis's files, one pension examiner noted his belief that Davis was "entirely unable to do anything useful."⁴⁵ It was harder to prove that other disabilities impacted the capacity for manual labor, especially when a veteran seemed outwardly able-bodied. Of course, Joshua Lawrence Chamberlain faced the dilemma of proving a nonvisible ailment while trying to convince the Pension Bureau's special examiner that he was, in fact, as disabled as he claimed. According to Peter Blanck's and Michael Millender's demographic study of pensions, easily proven or highly visible disabilities were more likely to receive a pension or a higher payout, while more nebulous ailments were more commonly rejected or offered lower rates.[46]

Black veterans faced yet more skepticism. Larry Logue and Peter Blanck's study of black veterans finds that the Pension Bureau favored ailments with "plentiful hospital evidence, such as intestinal disorders or the visibly inflamed joints of rheumatism, over maladies that were especially dependent on examining physicians' judgment, such as heart and respiratory diseases."[47] The case of Zechariah Davis bears this out. Davis served in the Seventh USCT and was hospitalized for an acute lung disease in 1864. Since then, he alleged, he had suffered recurring bouts of respiratory infection, as well as rheumatism and neuralgia. Four medical examinations later, surgeons concluded that Davis was at best slightly impaired but not incapable of manual labor. His application was rejected.[48] No doubt racist suspicions that black men were physically inferior and prone to disability, along with misgivings about their honesty and merit, played a role in determining their disability claims' authenticity.[49]

The Pension Bureau also adhered to the common beliefs that only certain disabilities had long-lasting or permanent symptoms, and that other ailments could, and perhaps *should*, be overcome. Though war wounds certainly held a cultural cachet, they were often interpreted as isolated events rather than lifelong realities. Nonvisible wounds like Chamberlain's or Nebraska senator Charles F. Manderson's were the most easily dismissed. Manderson, colonel of the Nineteenth Ohio Infantry, had been leading a charge at the Battle of Lovejoy Station when he was shot in the right side of his body. Physicians were unable to remove the ball, which caused spinal damage and resulted in temporary paralysis. Manderson was unable to return to his command, and he received a disability discharge in April 1865.[50] His pension application was approved that July. After the war, he found success as a lawyer and as a politician. Nearly twenty-five years later, Manderson underwent another surgical examination in hopes of raising his fifteen-dollar pension rating. The surgeon found that the injury threatened to cause paralysis, and that symptoms of the wound had increased. Pension examiners denied Manderson's claim, but Commissioner of Pensions James Tanner pushed it through anyway. The veteran was granted an increase and a considerable sum for arrears.[51]

Incredulous critics of the pension system were certain that Manderson could not be considered disabled. "The paralysis never came," the editors of the *Illustrated American* reminded readers. "Mr. Manderson's health was perfect, and his wound did not interfere with his indulging in dancing, an art in which he delighted."[52] The editors of Pennsylvania's *Harrisburg Patriot* put an even finer point on the matter, declaring, "Manderson is neither a disabled man nor a needy one.... He ought to be ashamed to be a beggar, a pensioner upon the bounty of men poorer than himself."[53] Secretary of the Interior John W. Noble agreed with critics and wrote Manderson a letter chastising him for accepting the pension payout. Likely humiliated by the imputation that he was something of a mercenary, Manderson returned his arrears payment and requested that his pension be lowered to its original rating.[54] While his wealth and power influenced his case, the senator's experience nonetheless demonstrated that postwar success was often interpreted as proof that a veteran was not actually disabled, regardless of his physical condition.

A disability could be entirely erased if it seemed that a veteran failed to meet standards of genteel manhood. Pvt. Murty Brennan had only served with the Forty-Eighth Pennsylvania for a few months when he was wounded during the Siege of Petersburg, receiving gunshot wounds to his left foot, left hip, and left arm, as well as a glancing shot in the forehead. Miraculously, Brennan recovered and served out the rest of the war with the Eighteenth Regiment of the Veteran Reserve Corps. Despite his obvious record of wartime disability—the Invalid Corps, after all, was exclusively for men disabled in the service—Brennan's pension application was rejected because it was unclear that his many wounds had left him disabled. When examined, surgeons noted that the former private did not have the "general appearance of a man of good habits." He was "'broken' for his age, no doubt due to his occupation & habits—not disabled by wounds or injuries."[55] Though the surgeons eventually suggested that Brennan deserved at least a small pension, Pension Bureau referee N. F. Graham rejected the ruling. Having never laid eyes on Murty Brennan, Graham stated definitively, "It is my opinion that the claimant is not disabled in any degree."[56] Despite his many bullet wounds, Murty Brennan ceased being a disabled veteran when it seemed as though he was a poor excuse for a man.

When a soldier failed to convince the Pension Bureau he was deserving, his next step was to appeal to his federal representatives. Seeking congressmen's assistance for pension problems became so common in the 1880s that one member of the House of Representatives recalled receiving fifty letters a week on on the topic. Another representative estimated that handling pension claims made up the majority of his congressional career.[57] Personal pension bills, like any other piece of legislation, required the signature of the president to take effect. Signing such bills had not been a concern to the Republican presidents preceding Grover Cleveland—none of his predecessors had vetoed a single pension bill. Even so, Cleveland considered these private bills symbolic of the pension system's endemic corruption.⁵⁸

Cleveland, a lifelong Democrat, had avoided conscription in 1863 by securing a Polish immigrant to serve as a substitute. In addition, the president was generally ambivalent about the war and its causes.⁵⁹ His feelings on veterans' rights were equally lukewarm. The president believed that the massive Grand Army of the Republic lobby exerted undue influence and helped to push through unworthy private pension bills. Its power seemed a holdover of preceding Republican administrations' corruption. Cleveland knew better than to blackball Union veterans wielding such electoral power, but he vehemently opposed the massive government spending that went into pensions. Republicans' and veterans' sense of entitlement irritated him.

Cleveland had installed his own Democratic commissioner of pensions, John C. Black, a Medal of Honor winner and veteran. Still, the president was unable to exert much control over the disbursement of funds under the existing laws.⁶⁰ The stacks of private pension bills on his desk awaiting signatures provided the opportunity for Cleveland to not only prove his commitment to exorcising fraud from the system, but also to send a message about who was and was not worthy of a pension. The veto messages, of course, reflected the important political realities of Cleveland's presidency. He was a Democratic president waging war against a Republican Congress and powerhouse Republican lobbying groups like the Grand Army of the Republic.⁶¹ Rather than simply rejecting the legislation, Cleveland used his vetoes to send larger cultural messages about disability and manhood. As president, he held ultimate power over the fate of a veteran's pension claim, and he wielded it to combat fraud and legitimize the idea that immoral former soldiers posed a looming threat.

The case of Abraham Griggs, the unfortunate soldier from this chapter's opening story, is a particularly useful example. Griggs's pension application follows the common narrative of a true soldier broken by war, and a man who desired to be productive though encumbered by impairment. "I was as sound as a dollar when I enlisted," wrote Griggs in a pension affidavit in 1891, "I was examined in a nude state, I had no rheumatism or other trouble, I was the strongest in this county before I enlisted."⁶² During the one year and four months of his service, Griggs's unit was present at thirty engagements, including Cedar Mountain, Thoroughfare Gap, Second Manassas, and Fredericksburg. It was after Fredericksburg that Griggs began to suffer from rheumatism. "I was in the battle of Fredericksburg on duty. I done my duty, never was off, from my enlistment until that Battle," the veteran insisted.⁶³ But after the battle, as the regiment camped in the cold and wet conditions of December in Virginia, Griggs's extremities grew painful and swollen. His condition soon became so severe that he was unable to grip his sword or mount his horse. Griggs tried to work through the pain, even going without socks or boots when his legs were too swollen, but he eventually was sent to Harewood Hospital in Washington, DC. After some time in Harewood, Griggs was transferred to his home state of New Jersey for further treatment.

His real troubles began at United States General Hospital in Newark. Several doctors, perhaps believing that work was a manful treatment for imprecise ailments, began to require Griggs and his fellow patients to perform manual labor around the hospital. Griggs and several others refused. "Dr. Taylor and Dr. Mills got angry at me in the last hospital I was in, they wanted me to work, to clean and sweep up and I refused to do it, they put me and ten or eleven others in the Guard House a couple of days because we wouldn't saw wood and clean up," Griggs explained to a pension clerk. Frustrated with these insubordinate patients, the doctors discharged all of them, but not before noting on each and every discharge form that the soldiers were lazy, worthless, and, in Griggs's case, fat. Those words became President Cleveland's deciding factor in vetoing the private bill.

Undeterred, Griggs reapplied for a pension in 1891. This time a special examiner questioned him. Griggs forthrightly explained that he had worked as a farmhand after his discharge, though recurring bouts of rheumatism had kept him from work several weeks a year. "I could do a pretty fair day's work at times," Griggs explained, "but I have been laid up at times, I couldn't cradle grain nor bend down to bind sheaves."[64] He also revealed that he had struggled with alcohol, admitting to drinking "a good deal of whisky" up to the late 1870s. Moreover, he addressed the allegations of the doctors who had discharged him: "I was no stouter in the Newark Hospital than now, no, my brain was not affected, I was not an imbecile nor any thing like it." He also spoke directly to the implication of malingering: "If [the doctor] thought that nothing was the matter why didn't he send me back to my Regiment?"[65]

The Pension Bureau special examiner, R. M. McMorris, could not help but agree with Griggs. "I cannot see why, if nothing was the matter with him, that he was kept eight months," McMorris stated, "and why he was not returned to his Regiment."[66] Even so, the examiner still doubted the veteran's character. Despite evidence that Griggs had served with his regiment for over a year without incident, McMorris noted, "I am inclined to think he was not what is called a good soldier." Instead, the bureau representative gave more weight to the allegations of malingering lodged by the doctors at the Newark hospital. It seemed impossible for Griggs to have been a good soldier if respected medical authorities had accused him of sloth and insubordination. As for the legitimacy of Griggs's disability, McMorris was equally skeptical. "I noticed in driving that he does not have use of his right hand," McMorris admitted, but the examiner still insisted that Griggs was only slightly disabled. This time, Griggs finally secured support, earning arrears and a twelve-dollar monthly pension. He didn't have long to enjoy his success—he died the next year.[67]

Griggs's case demonstrates the difficulty veterans faced in requesting government assistance. In spite of allegations from the press and president that pensions were hastily and carelessly pushed through Congress and the Pension Bureau, Griggs's case shows just how exacting the pension application process could be.[68] Though the veteran pointed to his good health prior to the war, his disability since the war, and his unmarred service in his cavalry unit, he faced allegations that challenged his manhood. Doctors described him as lazy, flabby, and "worthless." The implication that Griggs was an inferior man was the only evidence needed to prove he had been a malingerer. When Griggs's private pension bill arrived on the president's desk, the case seemed symbolic of the fraud Cleveland believed plagued the system. And so the president took the opportunity to shame cowards. After all, Griggs was not a true Union veteran, but a pathetic fraud who had falsified his disability to escape the war, then tried to con the United States government to get a handout.

In Abraham Griggs's case, charges of malingering supplied Cleveland with clear-cut justification for a veto. In other cases, though, the president had to probe the bill more thoroughly to determine the claimant's worth. Though he likely wouldn't have appreciated the comparison, Cleveland and the clerks at the Pension Bureau shared similar beliefs about worthiness. As we have seen, applications from men who displayed (or were accused of) weakness or unsoldierly behavior and those whose disabilities did not fit preconceived parameters were often met with criticism from the bureau. In a private bill, they were likely candidates for a presidential veto.

Cleveland shared the popular skepticism that certain ailments were disabling, especially when symptoms were not explicitly tied to the original wound. Even when veterans had well-documented war traumas, the president sometimes remained unconvinced of secondary complications or chronic symptoms. Many such cases were brought by widows, who needed to explicitly tie their husbands' deaths to their war service. For instance, Annie Owen applied for a pension in 1882, arguing that her husband's multiple wartime wounds and illnesses caused his 1876 death from "neuralgia of the heart." Mortimer B. Owen, second lieutenant in the Fifty-Seventh

Pennsylvania, had been wounded with shell fragments in the leg and side at Malvern Hill, and he had also suffered from remittent fever, diarrhea, chronic bronchitis, and acute dysentery, all within a ten-month period.

Comrades and physicians all testified that Owen's suffering in the army had changed him, and that he had never recovered his previous state of health. Nevertheless, Cleveland remained dubious. Owen had never applied for a pension, Cleveland pointed out, and his wife waited nearly a decade after his death to make an application. Moreover, Cleveland argued that the widow could not prove that her husband's heart disease was related to his wartime ailments. "If the wounds were received as described here," the president wrote in his veto of Mrs. Owen's bill, "there is certainly no necessary connection between them and the death fourteen years afterward from neuralgia of the heart."[69] It certainly seems possible to a modern reader—and it seemed perfectly logical to the veteran's doctors and loved ones—that Owen was experiencing physical manifestations of a stress response. But Cleveland rejected any linkage between a war wound, camp diseases, and a postwar heart condition.

Republican senator William Joyce Sewell, himself a Union veteran, pushed back against Cleveland's assessment of Owen's case. Sewell, member of the Senate Committee on Pensions, accused Cleveland of cherry-picking his evidence and ignoring all of the numerous testimonials supporting Mrs. Owen's claim. The testimony that Cleveland favored, Sewell alleged, "is not based upon facts . . . is wholly negative in its character, and is merely the substance of the opinions of three or four men who have not and do not offer a single proof of their own knowledge." The senator then supplied statements from eighteen different doctors, comrades, and acquaintances that backed Owen's claim. Further, Sewell and the committee were appalled that Cleveland would use Owen's failure to apply for a pension during his lifetime against him. After all, shouldn't that delay please the president, who strove to keep pension payouts down? "The Committee," wrote Sewell, "think that this refusal on the soldier's part to become a recipient of Government bounty reflects honor upon his manhood and does credit to his patriotism."[70]

Cleveland was also skeptical of mental illness, rejecting claims that it could stem from combat. During his first term in office, he vetoed eleven cases concerning widows of disabled veterans who had committed suicide in the decades after their discharge. Most often, these cases were dismissed because Cleveland argued that the applicants could not definitively prove that the war had triggered the veterans' suicide. Jane Potts sought a pension after her husband, Noah, formerly a private in the Seventh Illinois Cavalry, drowned himself. Noah Potts had been a prisoner of the Confederacy in Georgia's notorious Andersonville Prison. According to comrade Nealy Woods, Potts had been a strong and capable soldier, but after his release from Andersonville, "he was a skeleton on account of hardships he had endured [and] ... he believed his bones were rotten." Woods also testified that Potts's mind "dwelt on his imprisonment, and it was difficult to draw it to any other subject, and that he was very absent-minded."[71] Cleveland, however, chose to believe the special examiner, who had determined that it was Jane Potts's nagging, not memories of his abuse in Andersonville, that had driven Noah Potts to suicide. "This evidence," Cleveland wrote, "reconciles me to the conclusion ... that the military service and prison experience of the deceased were in no manner connected with his death."[72]

Cleveland was similarly unsympathetic to soldiers who overdosed on opiates they used to manage pain. When her husband died of a morphine overdose, Anna Mertz applied for a pension. Charles Mertz had suffered from intense bouts of diarrhea as well as terrible pain from severe catarrh, which he "constantly attributed to his army service." He self-administered morphine to combat his chronic pain, but Cleveland dismissed the connection: "I do not think the death of the soldier was so related to his military service as to entitle his widow to a pension."[73] Tamezan Ball's son, Augustus F. Caldicott, overdosed on laudanum while slowly and painfully dying of a lung condition contracted during his time with the Seventy-Fifth New York.[74] The young man was pensioned for the lung disease, so the Pension Bureau already accepted the condition's veracity. According to the physicians who had prescribed the laudanum, Caldicott died because "his intensified sufferings compelled him to take a dose that proved too much for him in his enfeebled condition."[75] But Cleveland saw no connection between the soldier's death and the suffering caused by the condition. In addition, the president did little to mask his disdain for men who turned to drugs for pain relief: "I see nothing unjust or unfair in holding that if a pensioner is sick and through ignorance or design takes laudanum without the direction or regulation of a physician the Government should not be held responsible for the consequences."[76]

The case of Eliza Smith and her late husband, Clinton, caused a bit of a public outcry, at least in the couple's home state of Indiana. "It is enough to make an honest man's blood boil," seethed the editors of the *Indianapolis Journal*.[77] Eliza Smith had applied for a continuation of her husband's benefits after he died in 1884, most likely of a morphine overdose. Clinton Smith had been with his regiment, the Eighty-Fourth Indiana, during the Battle of Chickamauga, when he was shot in the left arm. That he was wounded at Chickamauga was hardly surprising—the Eighty-Fourth Indiana suffered a more than 35 percent casualty rate within a few short hours of fighting.[78] Field surgeons had performed an excision rather than an amputation, which meant removing an inch and a half of Smith's humerus, leaving his arm practically useless. The remaining portions of bone became infected and slowly began to die, continually spitting shards into his arm.

To make matters worse, the wound itself never healed, remaining in a state of near-constant infection and drainage.[79] These infections dramatically affected Smith's overall health. "I have seen him writhe scores of times and moan most bitterly," testified a friend, "til I thought the man would take his life to end his sufferings." Smith testified in one pension application that the wound had "gathered and broke, or been lanced [for drainage] sixty eight times."[80] Smith was prescribed morphine to curb his intense pain. In 1884, while staying with a friend, the veteran suffered an attack of pain and asked for morphine. Apparently unable to find any, he retreated to his bedroom. By the next afternoon, he was dead. It was presumed, though not proven, that he had located the drug and subsequently overdosed.

Eliza Smith later applied to Congress to continue receiving her late husband's pension. The bill passed, but it required Cleveland's signature to be enacted. The president was unmoved by Clinton Smith's story. He focused on the man's use of morphine, not on his pain: "His family physician testified that . . . he was in the habit of taking morphine in large doses, and that at times he was intemperate, especially when suffering from his wound. It seems it would establish a very bad precedent to allow a pension upon the facts developed in this case."[81] To Cleveland, the use of any amount of pain medication, even when prescribed, proved weakness. Regardless of the reasons for Smith's morphine use, his overdose demonstrated that he had been "intemperate" and thus unworthy of support. The *Indianapolis Journal* was appalled: "The President affects to believe that the deceased died from an overdose of morphine, self-administered, and intimates that it might have been due to intemperance. This is a gratuitous assumption and insult; but even if it were true it would not lessen the force or merit of the claim."[82]

President Cleveland's vetoes reflect more than the desire to moderate governmental expenditures. Rather, Cleveland latched onto evidence that veterans were addicts, cowards, and beggars. His motivation was ostensibly to protect the pension system for the truly deserving soldiers, but the subtext of his language in the veto messages suggests moral judgments about masculinity and veteran status. The veto messages show strict boundaries between worth and deviancy. A man like Clinton Smith might have been a brave soldier during his time in the Eighty-Fourth Indiana, but his decision to turn to morphine negated his earlier reputation. Such weakness revealed a veteran incapable of manfully bearing the necessary pains of war. Cleveland argued that the pension roll should be sacred. He believed the only way to ensure that government support remained a mark of gratitude and honor was to "exclude perversion as well as insure a liberal and generous application of grateful and benevolent designs."[83] In this scenario, strictly policing the boundaries between able and disabled, worthy and unworthy, kept the pension free from the "perversion" of the mercenary, deserter, and malingerer. The Cleveland vetoes resulted from a contentious Democratic presidency with an opposition Congress, but they also reflected and amplified public debates about what it meant to be a true disabled soldier of Union.

Late nineteenth-century debates over the pension system concerned more than trimming the federal budget or making public welfare more effective; these debates dealt with what kinds of men deserved the support of the state. Disability pensions were ostensibly designed for all soldiers wounded or sickened during the war. Yet those who failed to adhere to the expectations of idealized manhood or who lived with ailments outside the Pension Bureau's definition of disability found themselves without support. Moreover, such veterans were labeled immoral and unmanly. Categorizing troublesome old soldiers as mercenaries, deserters, malingerers, and frauds rejected them and removed them from the ranks of legitimate Union veterans.

Troublesome soldiers in the pension system were rhetorically disconnected, removed from the roll of honor through accusations of insufficient manhood and exaggerated impairments. These men were pilloried in the press, excluded from national celebrations of the true Union soldier, cut off from the national gratitude promised at the end of the war. But while such veterans were symbolically separated, other soldiers were actually separated—not just from the ranks of their comrades, but from the rest of society. Veterans committed to asylums and labeled insane were forced to live separately from family and community. As we have seen, soldiers with nonvisible disabilities struggled to get the acknowledgment and support of society; those with truly invisible mental wounds faced an even more uncertain future. And when a soldier sunk into insensibility, war trauma radiated outward, affecting even those who had never set foot on the field of battle.

CHAPTER 6

The Long, Long Years of Misery

Over the course of four decades, Lizzie Wilson McReynolds sent letter after letter to the superintendents of the St. Elizabeths Hospital in Washington, DC, a treatment facility and home for hundreds of mentally ill Union soldiers and veterans. McReynolds wrote for information about her brother, John Wilson, a veteran and permanent inmate of the asylum. Sister and brother had been separated since their parents had sent John to St. Elizabeths, and hundreds of miles lay between them. In her correspondence, McReynolds expressed her longing to see John again, fussed over his care and his access to little luxuries like cigars and candy, and schemed about his possible transfer to a facility closer to home. She also pondered the nature of John's disability. "I think with a pang [of] when he was the best of Brothers and was one of the brightest young men in the Neighborhood," she wrote in one letter, "and now he is a Wreck and for what[?]" Lizzie answered her own question, perhaps as an uncertain afterthought. In her cramped hand, she added the words "to free the country" in the small space between the lines.[1]

Forty years after the Civil War's end, Lizzie McReynolds was still struggling to come to terms with her brother's disability. Her letters to the asylum were not only a way to gather information about her brother, but also an outlet for her meditations on the nature and reality of war-related mental illness. Like many touched by war trauma, McReynolds felt helpless. She could not fully comprehend John's condition, overcome the distance separating them, or even ensure his comfort. In her correspondence, she challenged her powerlessness by demanding the superintendent's time and attention and micromanaging her brother's care. Mostly, though, the letters became a safe place for McReynolds to contemplate her own feelings about her sibling's state. "Poor, poor John," she lamented in one letter, "he was witty, smart, and handsome, and [now] the long, long years of misery and darkened mind. I won't write any more about it."[2]

Suffering is both individual and social.[3] While war trauma immediately impacted soldiers, it also radiated outward and affected loved ones. This was certainly true for soldiers who bore physical wounds—Joshua and Fanny Chamberlain's marriage was a powerful example of how one war wound could have effects both individual and interpersonal. In this chapter, we explore how wounded minds were experienced on both an individual and relational level. War trauma rendered disabled soldiers and their families powerless in a variety of ways. Some institutionalized soldiers worried about their chances at future success and had to hope others—family members, guardians, and physicians—might secure their release so that they could rehabilitate their manhood through work. Violent manifestations of mental illness and the distance imposed by the asylum separated families from one another, making it impossible for relations to carry out culturally prescribed roles and actions. Wives could not care for mentally ill soldiers, and institutionalized husbands were unable to provide for their families. Mothers and fathers died without their sons at their bedside. War trauma made it difficult for many family members, like Lizzie McReynolds, to even come to terms with what had turned their soldiers into wrecks. This multidimensional trauma defied the boundaries of war, invaded domestic spaces, and extracted an emotional toll on veterans and their loved ones little by little over the years.

Recently, historians have debated the existence of combat-related mental illness in Civil War soldiers. The conversation has often centered on the efficacy of using post-traumatic stress disorder (PTSD), a modern diagnosis unknown to mid-nineteenth-century Americans, to understand psychological reactions to the Civil War. Several scholars have done a great deal to identify the existence of soldiers' and veterans' trauma. Others have rightly noted that diagnoses like PTSD are rooted in the social and cultural context of the twentieth century, not the nineteenth.[4] The social model of disability also argues that disability is socially and culturally constructed. As such, mental disabilities can only be understood within their time- and culture-specific context. Here, I do not use the term *PTSD*—following the precedent set by Diane Miller Sommerville, I use the term *war trauma*—nor do I spend time trying to identify historical subjects' diagnoses. Determining whether soldiers' symptoms fit a modern diagnosis, or are better explained by another diagnosis or underlying disorder, traps us in the medical model of disability. In addition, these endeavors do little to help us understand the ways in which affected soldiers and their families made sense of and coped with the reality of mental illness.[5]

Instead, this chapter explores the stories of soldiers, veterans, and their families as told in the patient case files of the New York State Lunatic Asylum at Utica (Utica), the Willard Asylum for the Chronic Insane (Willard), both located in upstate New York, and St. Elizabeths Hospital in Washington, DC.[6] In each case, someone—the soldier himself, his family, or his physicians—identified the war as a cause or a precipitating event in the course of a veteran's illness. Patient case files contain the medical records of a soldier's or veteran's war trauma, but they also include any material relevant to the person receiving treatment. In many cases, attendants and doctors glued patients' letters to the pages of ledgers or tucked them into their file folders. For soldiers and family members separated by geographic and emotional distance, and powerless against a force they struggled to comprehend, these communications became a space where they could grapple with the complexities of mental illness, pine for a loved one, or beg for release from the asylum.[7] Taken together, the case files, correspondence, and other documents offer a unique look into the lives of those living with war-related mental disability. The cases described here are anecdotal and not necessarily representative of larger trends. Even so, they paint a compelling emotional portrait of the ways combat trauma affected some soldiers and families even decades after the war's end.

The Soldiers

When Daniel Folsom was sent to the New York State Asylum for the Insane in Utica, his family and physicians agreed that the war had caused of his troubles.[8] Folsom had been a hardworking young tinsmith before his enlistment, and he was in good health for the majority of his service. The previous eighteen months had been arduous for the Sixteenth New York Infantry. In May 1862, Folsom's company had been caught in a small but fierce engagement at Eltham's Landing during the Peninsula Campaign. "In this battle," recalled regimental historian William Thompson, "the enemy practiced the most barbarous brutality upon our wounded." The corpse of one soldier was found with its throat cut, while another slain man had "not less than seven bayonet stabs on his body." According to Thompson, Confederate soldiers had also stripped the bodies of dead and wounded New Yorkers, stealing their clothing and other possessions. The historian hardly had words for the conduct of the brutal skirmish: "Comment is unnecessary."[9] Still, Folsom served well under such conditions, only showing "unusual excitement" during the regiment's service at Fredericksburg that winter.

But when Folsom returned home in the spring of 1863, his behavior became erratic. At first, he focused on work and opened his own tin shop. Soon, though, he began to wander away from his business for long periods. When the draft occurred in his hometown he panicked, fearing he might be sent back into battle. "This state of excitement," noted his intake physician, "left him two weeks in a depressed condition, despondent, suicidal—attempted his life by cutting himself."[10] Unable to ensure his son's safety, Folsom's father brought him to the asylum. Whether his company's experience at Eltham's Landing or some other stressor had sparked Folsom's breakdown can't be known, but the doctor who conducted Folsom's intake scribbled "excitement of battle" as the cause for the young man's mental state.[11]

Daniel Folsom did not improve quickly in the asylum. He told doctors that he was but a "crazy good for nothing fellow" and asked attendants to put him out of his misery. Paranoid and suspicious, he focused on getting out of Utica and home to northern New York. His only chances were either to recover quickly and fully enough to please the doctors, or to convince his father to remove him from the hospital. In March 1864, Folsom wrote his sister in hopes that she would plead his case to their father. The letter, and the sibling bond it symbolized, gave Folsom a safe place to reflect on his situation. Mostly, he yearned for home. He had only been home from the war for a few months before they had been separated again. "I wish you would come and see me, if nothing more," Folsom told his sister. He also inquired after family members, stating, "I have a kind of an akin to get home and see all of the folks."[12]

He had other reasons for wanting to get out. Staying longer in the institution, Folsom worried, could destroy his chances to establish himself as a tradesman. He was losing precious time, and he doubtless feared that the stigma of madness would follow him. "Iff I stay here any longer the world will be a blank and I really think there is a chance for me yet," he wrote. Folsom hoped his father might get him released so he could start working again. The possibility of getting back to work would be a recovery in itself, rehabilitating the veteran's identity as a productive and self-reliant man—rather than a confined invalid. Still, he acknowledged that might not be possible. "It is very hard to be confined so long," Folsom confessed to his sister. But he then resumed the submissiveness of the patient, stating, "Perhaps it is all for my good."[13]

Gregory Toombs, a private in the Seventy-Second New York, had a similar experience, but one with a striking exception. While Folsom asked his family to retrieve him from the asylum, Toombs took it on himself to escape. Gregory Toombs had been wounded during the Peninsula Campaign, but he stayed in the ranks and served well until the Battle of Gettysburg in July 1863. He was sent to the Government Hospital for the Insane just days after the battle, then discharged from the service disabled. Toombs returned home to upstate New York a few weeks later. In September, his father delivered him to Utica; the elder Toombs was worried about an apparent change in his son's character. The soldier was anxious and manic, and he swore. (Perhaps the last behavior was more a symptom of soldiering than of an unsettled mind.)[14] Gregory Toombs wanted to get back to the army, and after just a few days in the asylum, he hopped the fence and traveled to Albany. There, he later reported, he had intended to ask the governor for a commission.

Toombs returned to the asylum voluntarily but escaped again after the new year. He had been a student prior to his enlistment, and he was so anxious to leave Utica and finish his education that he took advantage of a moment of freedom while working on the hospital grounds. He returned to school, but his life did not return to normal. Instead, his former friends treated him with disdain and suspicion. "Says he went right home to friends and soon commenced going to school," noted a doctor, "but he found all the people in the neighborhood & his fellow scholars in particular treat him with much reserve and it was evident to him they suspected his sanity." Toombs grew nervous. He had believed that he was recovered, but his staring classmates made him doubt his assessment of his own mental health. Toombs had seized a bit of control over his fate based on his understanding of his own body, but like Daniel Folsom, he resigned himself to accept his physicians' authority. The soldier again returned to Utica, where he was "willing to remain until pronounced well by faculty."[15] An official declaration of recovery might help him reenter society, but it came at a cost. While his doctor noted that Toombs was slowly recovering, Toombs also seemed to be suffering. After he was hurt in an altercation with another patient, he became depressed, then declared that he should never have returned.

Some thirteen years after he was discharged, Toombs wrote to John P. Gray, then superintendent of Utica, asking for the exact dates of his time at the asylum. The veteran wanted to bolster his application for a pension increase. Looking back, he was frustrated at the disparity between the laxness of his wartime physicians and the thoroughness of pension examiners. "I wish to God," he complained, "they had had as sharp a set at the other end of the performance, ie, when they discharged me from the U.S. Insane Asylum after my being there only three weeks."[16] His quick discharge,

Toombs believed, had made it appear as though his later problems were unrelated to his wartime illness. "The Govt. always trys to lay the cause of disease on to something else beside military service," he complained to Gray. Toombs insisted that the Civil War had negatively affected his life. "I was wounded twice & my military record is clear & am sure the war made a great difference with me," he wrote, adding, "Lost the same as twelve or fourteen years by it."[17]

Driven by homesickness and anxiety over their future prospects, both Gregory Toombs and Daniel Folsom were intent on getting out of the asylum. They worried that institutionalization would leave a lifelong stain on their character. Worse, they feared they might never recover at all. Benjamin Ellis was also anxious to leave the hospital and find employment, but he was afraid that he could not trust his mind. Like Toombs, Ellis worried he could not understand his own condition. Ellis had been in St. Elizabeths for two years when he wrote to his uncle and sought advice on whether he could, or should, attempt to return home and seek work. The veteran worried he could not be trusted to behave properly or to assess his own health. "I do not know whether my condition would be improved by my return," Ellis told his uncle, "& I feel as if I did not know for myself as well as some of my friends who are older & more experienced." He wanted to come home. But he also admitted, "I feel as if there was some obstruction in my way perhaps I am not entirely well of Insanity."[18]

Although wounded at the Siege of Port Hudson, Ellis had served for the duration of the war with no signs of mental distress. After his discharge, he reenlisted in the regular army and served for an additional three years before being sent to St. Elizabeths in 1868. By 1870, Ellis was showing signs of worry over his future. "I have been here over 2 years & have tried to be contented," Ellis wrote to his uncle. The soldier wanted to leave, but he was also terribly afraid that he would be useless outside of the hospital, or that his illness would worsen. "I suppose it [is] thought here that I am incapable of earning my living by my daily labor, if that is the case it would be better for me to continue here," he wrote, "but if [I] could come home I would try to work for a subsistence."[19] Ellis asked his uncle to help him create a plan for his future, especially because they would need to present the doctors with a clear proposal for his release. He was afraid to hope for a release, but clearly he wanted to be home, or at least among loved ones. "Please give my love to all friends and relatives," Ellis wrote. "I do not have any hopes of getting home now, may the Lord help me in my lonely life."[20]

Writing to his family and friends at home in the winter of 1865, Charles Danielson echoed the desire to leave the asylum and start working. Danielson had served with the 146th New York for only a few months before his discharge. His release from service followed his arrest as a deserter, at which time he was found insensible.[21] After a few months in the Utica facility, Danielson assured loved ones that he was comfortable. But he also said that he missed them and was ready to be released. "I want you to . . . make Prepp-preations to get me from this building as soon as possible," he instructed family and friends. A musician, Danielson was eager to find a traveling troupe with which to perform. He assured his family that he understood his place as a patient, but he also believed that he was getting well enough to leave: "I am happy here all through Life if [I] had not another home but I must come home soon and goo to work, I am getting well enough fast enough to brave it."[22]

Institutionalized soldiers and veterans were both isolated and powerless over their confinement. For these men, letters were more than an emotional link to loved ones. Correspondence was their only way of negotiating for a freedom that guardians and physicians alone could grant. Many asylum inmates asked their loved ones to help them secure a release so that they could get back to work. Productivity, the central feature differentiating the disabled pauper from the able-bodied man, seemed like the key to success-fully reentering society. This focus on work reflected nineteenth-century notions of pauperism and dependency. Moreover, it prefigured post–World War I reformers' efforts to use vocational training to rehabilitate soldiers in the belief that labor would "remasculinize" disabled veterans.[23] Yet asylum patients' letters also show that soldiers and veterans deferred to physicians' expertise and doubted their ability to assess their own minds, leaving them unsure they could successfully reintegrate into society. Gregory Toombs, for example, decided he was well enough to leave the hospital against orders and go back to school. Once there, the stares of his peers left him questioning his sanity. Could they see something he could not? The internalized sense of deviance and inferiority left soldiers like Toombs unsure they could ever adequately reconstruct their manhood through industrious living. Feelings of inadequacy also reinforced physicians' and guardians' power to determine a soldier's state of sanity or insanity.

Not all soldiers were quite so uncertain about their ability to rehabilitate their manhood. Robert Martin expressed no doubt that he was well and ready to leave the asylum. As a private in the 126th New York, Martin had suffered a severe bout of typhoid fever that made him confused and for-getful. His mental condition had continued to deteriorate after he returned home, and he remained in a similar state for months after his May 1863 commitment to Utica. The following February, Martin suddenly became lucid. He asked where he was and why he wasn't with his regiment, and he was much surprised to find himself in an institution rather than a parole camp. He had no memory of the preceding months. A few weeks later, Martin wrote to his parents asking them take him out of the asylum. He would improve more quickly, he believed, if he was allowed to get out and start working: "When I get home I think my strength will increase faster. *I want to get to work*. Do not love to be idle so much."[24]

Some soldiers had more immediate concerns than getting back into the workforce. Sailor Jeremiah Norris voiced desperation in a June 1863 letter to his brother: "If you love your Brother for gods sake get me out of here immediately." Norris had distinguished himself during a naval bombardment by picking up a live shell on the deck of the ship and flinging it into the water before it could explode onboard. During the same conflict, he had been struck in the head with a piece of spent shell. Afterward, Norris complained of "a darting pain passing from frontal to occipital region of head" that came with periods of "forgetfulness, confusion of ideas, false perceptions & wrong deductions."[25] He was discharged disabled, and on his journey home he attempted to drown himself. Norris was rescued, and he subsequently returned home depressed, listless, and uninterested in friends or surroundings. When the depression devolved into delusions, his family thought it best that he be treated in an asylum.

Norris's doctor dismissed out of hand his belief that the head wound had caused his condition. The physician instead concluded that the problem stemmed from chronic masturbation, and used a blistering plaster on the sailor's penis. It is little wonder Norris wanted to be out of the asylum. "You said that father would come after me as soon as Doc. Gray would say that I was well," he wrote to his brother. "He will never say that long as father will pay board here it is the object to keep patients here as long as he can." To drive the point home, Norris made his condition clear: "The doct. Blistered my p 4 times and I took hold of it and I thought it was going to rot off."[26] A few months later, Norris gave up on getting his father's intervention or his doctors' approval. He took his case into his own hands by escaping the asylum.

Aside from Benjamin Norris and his poor blistered penis, most soldiers aimed to get out of the asylum and back to work in the belief that labor would be rehabilitative. If they were no longer soldiers, work represented these veterans' greatest opportunity to cast off the stigma of madness and restore their manhood. Of course, that recovery required them to hold down a job. The case of Edgar Brown suggests what could happen to veterans who failed to stay productive. A shoemaker and veteran of Berdan's Sharpshooters,

Brown supported himself and his wife and son for decades after the war. But he began struggling with his mental health in his early forties. Whether he had experienced episodes of mental illness during the intervening postwar decades is not recorded, but his brother Franklin testified that Edgar's insanity stemmed from two war wounds.

In 1882, Edgar Brown stopped working, apparently unable to find decent employment. He moved in with his brother and was "non-self-supporting," relying on his brother's family for care. Edgar's state worsened in 1885; he experienced unexplained convulsions and became severely distressed. Franklin Brown had no choice but to take his brother to the Willard Asylum, explaining that Edgar had been "morose lately, & threatened suicide because he could not find work being a fine workman." When the admitting physicians asked Edgar to explain the many scars on his body, he said that his face had been cut "by the blow of [a] sabre of an enemy in the army, in the line of duty.... Also scar on the right side received while in army, by explo[sion] of a limber cart and [said] he was sick eight months afterward."[27] While in the asylum, Edgar Brown's health worsened, and within three weeks, he was dead.

Despite the dire prospects that institutionalized soldiers saw for themselves, there were positive endings. In fact, most of the men profiled here went on to have successful careers and, as far as the evidence shows, typical, perhaps even happy, lives. When Daniel Folsom wrote to his sister in 1864, he added a postscript: "I shall try and be a man."[28] He kept his word by reenlisting in the Union army upon his release from Utica, perhaps hoping to reaffirm his manhood through battle. When the war ended, he mustered out as a first lieutenant in a New York regiment.[29] Folsom returned to upstate New York, worked as a tinsmith, married, and fathered six daughters.[30] Robert Martin returned to his prior career as a bookkeeper and worked for the same Hudson, New York, bank for nearly half a century.[31] Gregory Toombs, too, had a long career among the ranks of veterans with patronage jobs in the U.S. Post Office.[32]

Such comparatively positive endings are an important reminder that war trauma was not simple or static. Each of these soldiers and veterans experienced mental illness profound enough to warrant a stay in an asylum, but they lived typical lives after their release. This is not evidence that their trauma was somehow less severe or that they "overcame" disability. What these men's experiences do suggest is that combat trauma in the Civil War era did not fit strict categories of sanity and insanity. Certainly, as several scholars argue and as we will see later in this chapter, some traumatized soldiers and veterans were unable to live seemingly typical lives. Some were permanently institutionalized, and others even chose to end their own lives.[33] Yet Folsom, Martin, and Toombs demonstrate that trauma could be just one element of a veteran's life, rather than its defining element. How many other Union veterans shared the experience of bouts of anguish followed by years of stability? If some traumatized soldiers also led more or less typical lives, might it have been possible that war trauma was a more common experience, one that only rose to the surface of the historical record when at its most acute? These cases are too few to provide solid answers. But at the very least, they offer some evidence for the existence of war trauma in veterans who gave the appearance of health.

Soldiers and veterans institutionalized for war-related mental illness used their letters home to express homesickness and longing for freedom. The most common aims for these men were getting out and getting to work. War-traumatized soldiers believed that maintaining productivity was the only way they could rehabilitate their manhood. This notion echoed the approaches to disability used by war-related institutions ranging from the Invalid Corps to the Pension Bureau. For some, this rehabilitation plan worked. For others, it wasn't possible. And for the families of those who remained in the asylum, the emotional toll of living apart subsumed worries about productivity.

The Families

In their letters home, institutionalized soldiers and veterans focused on immediate and personal problems. But the letters sent from home to the asylum show that trauma affected more than a soldier or veteran himself. Those missives, when combined with snippets and stories from patient case files and pension documents, make it clear that war trauma also had immediate and often severe consequences for families. Wives struggled to act as caretakers for children and husbands while also assuming the role of provider. Soldiers lashed out as their illness manifested itself in violence directed toward those closest to them. For others kept apart by the asylum, the trauma was in the separation.[34] In their testimony, we see how families torn apart and struggling to understand the nature of combat trauma carried the emotional scars of a war they did not fight.

War trauma upended domestic order and strained traditional family roles. When a soldier returned home changed, his family members often had to rearrange their lives around his illness. Relatives had to learn to take on new roles, and wives most often bore the brunt of this new reality. Wives had to expand their existing role as caretaker to include the care of their dependent husbands. In addition, such women had little choice but to assume the additional role of provider. When Maria Kielhoffer's husband, Francis, returned from his service in the Thirty-Third New Jersey Infantry in the summer of 1865, she noticed changes in him immediately. A tailor, her husband had been healthy and of sound mind when he had enlisted in the Thirty-Third. After his war service, "he exhibited distinct signs of dementation, and suffered from scurvy, which affected his limbs." Though Francis returned to work quickly, he was unable to concentrate on his occupation, and the work he completed was poor. "The work he did had to be undone frequently, I would have to do it over, so as to pass inspection at the shop," Maria explained.[35]

When he eventually stopped working entirely, Maria tried to have Francis do work around the house, but he lost track of what he had been asked to do. After asking him to chop firewood, she discovered him half-heartedly hacking at the chopping stump instead of splitting wood. When she asked him to lay a new garden bed, she discovered him chatting to himself while digging and re-digging the same small hole. Francis's inability to work meant that Maria had no choice but to earn money to support the household. "His mental condition obliged me to do washing and ironing to support him and our children as well as myself," she explained. Even as she tried to complete her work, Francis cut Maria's clotheslines, meaning she had to rewash all the clients' laundry—no small task. The manifestation of Francis's disability meant that Maria had to do her own housework, take on extra work to pay the bills, and do Francis's work as well.[36]

Harriet Zane's husband was already an inmate of St. Elizabeths when she wrote to the institution in 1877. Rather than inquiring about Joseph Zane's well-being, Harriet expressed concern that the superintendent might send the man home. "I have no place for him," she explained, "I have no home for myself, only just where I work, and that is from place to place." Having effectively lost her husband during the war, Harriet Zane had little choice but to significantly restructure her life. Without a partner to help provide for the family, she had resorted to sending her five children to live with others. To support herself, Harriet worked several jobs. "I have done the hardest kind of work such as housecleaning washing and all kinds of laborious work," she wrote to the superintendent, "and now [I] am broke down." It's not that she didn't love her husband or wish that they could be together again, she insisted. In truth, reunion was impossible if Joseph could not contribute to the household.[37]

Women sometimes had an even more pressing reason to have the soldiers and veterans in their family committed: violence. It's often unclear why exactly a veteran became violent at home, but in their reports to hospital staff, family members described the behavior as an extension of a physical wound or the strain of warfare. In some cases, mothers became the target of soldiers' outbursts. Geoffrey Johnson experienced periods of depression before the war but began having "epileptic fits" while serving in the Union army. These episodes became more severe after he returned home. Sometimes, during a fit of "maniacal paroxysm," he became "violent to his family . . . &c drew [a] knife on his mother." Johnson turned the knife on himself in a suicide attempt, but his parents intervened in time and decided their son had to be hospitalized. Another veteran, army surgeon Isaiah Seaborn, walked back to upstate New York after he was taken prisoner during the Battle of Gettysburg and released by his captors. At first, Seaborn seemed unusually quiet and confused, but he soon became wild and delusional. He "threatened his mother's life, said she was not his mother, and endeavored to seize a gun to shoot 'that woman.'" Seaborn did not hurt his mother, but he instead turned his attention toward killing himself until his uncles interceded and had him committed at Utica.[38]

Wives were also vulnerable. Michael Mitchell, wounded in the head at Fredericksburg, alternately threatened to murder his wife by slitting her throat with a butcher knife or shooting her. When his head hurt, he made "threats of violence to any & all members of his family."[39] Jacob Kyle was "irritated by slight causes," and he flew into rages "so violent at times as to break and destroy everything within his reach." When he was in this state, he lashed out at anyone who dared to come near him. "He is dangerous to be at large," the intake doctor noted, continuing, "At short intervals he becomes violent attempting to kill his wife or son or friends, breaking everything he can get his hands on. Throwing dishes at his family while at their meals." The family could not endure the constant barrage of abuse, so Kyle was committed to the Willard Asylum.[40] Maria Kielhoffer, who had struggled to care for her husband, Francis, at home, eventually committed him to the Essex County Home for the Insane in Newark, New Jersey, when he became violent and threatened to kill her.[41]

Though women were often the most vulnerable to attack, everyone within the household could be at risk when a veteran raged. William Brenton, wounded in the head at Gettysburg, returned home delusional and paranoid. When his family tried to talk to him about his behavior, he threatened to burn the house down and kill the entire family.[42] Clinton Moore, formerly of the 144th New York, generally terrorized his family. He was brought to Utica after "drinking freely, abusing his family & threatening his wife's life." But Moore escaped. While he was home, he began "manifesting his old and dangerous tendencies," and his family was horrified by his renewed violence against them—his wife feared for her life, and he "whipped his children severely so one of them [was] obliged to leave home."⁴³ At one point, when a sheriff's deputy came to arrest him, Moore flung a large metal stove down the stairs at the officer. The constable, no doubt perturbed, described Moore to the asylum doctors as "3 parts ugly & 1 part crazy."⁴⁴ Even Robert Martin, the young man in Utica who went on to a long and respected career as a bookkeeper, had violent outbursts toward his family before his commitment. During one episode, Martin "struck his mother & little brother," then "attempted to gouge his father's eyes out."⁴⁵

If domestic disturbance and threats of violence demonstrate the most direct ways that war trauma affected families, the long separations accompanying institutionalization show the deep emotional toll a soldier's condition took on his loved ones. In their letters, family members grappled with the nature of their beloved's disability. They tried to come to terms with an impairment that lacked clear causation or outward signs yet was severe enough to merit commitment. Family members often expressed confused grief for a man that no longer existed, and they attempted to reconcile their memory of that man with the reality of the one now living in an institution.

In a letter to the superintendent of St. Elizabeths, Mary Ellis, sister of Benjamin Ellis, the veteran who wrote to his uncle hoping for a discharge, lamented her brother's altered future. Mary also asked that the superintendent release Benjamin; she hoped he might be able to find work outside of the institution. "I would like to have him where he could be happy & useful," she wrote, revealing her hopefulness. Perhaps if he lived with his parents and secured a pension, her brother could live happily enough with a small job. But Mary made it clear that while this was the best-case scenario, it was not what the family had expected for Benjamin's future. "When he went in the army he bid fair to be a useful man," she wrote. She added, "His intellect was fair, he was likely to be one of the best scholars in the school where he attended."⁴⁶ Now, Mary only hoped he might be able to live at home where they could care for him themselves.

The case files at St. Elizabeths, a residential asylum that released few profoundly disabled soldiers, are particularly fat with letters from heartsick loved ones. Family members wrote to the superintendents seeking information about men who had been hospitalized for years, even decades. In some cases, communication from the asylum was so infrequent that families literally had no idea whether their veterans were alive or dead. James Wright wrote in 1886 about his brother, "Please inform as to the condition of Johnithan Wright if he still lives he was an old soldier."⁴⁷ In 1879, Minnie Flenniken inquired whether her brother Samuel was living or dead. "Will you please tell me if my Brother Samuel Whiteside is he still living and is he no better?" she asked Dr. Godding. "Does he known anything if I were to see him do you think he would know me?" She added an indication of her—and Samuel's—pain: "Oh, I want to see him so much. is the ball still in his spine and don't you think it could be removed?"[48]

A farmer from Indiana named Caleb Moncrief wrote to Godding in 1886 asking after his father, John T. Moncrief, veteran of the Eleventh Illinois and resident of St. Elizabeths. The young man likely had no real memories of the man, who had gone off to war when Caleb was only three years old. "I want to now if at iney tim he ever ses eny thing about his family," the younger Moncrief asked. He added: "is he getting much gray[?]" The letter is brief, but it clearly indicates that Caleb Moncrief spent time wondering about his father. Did the elder Moncrief have any thoughts of his family in Indiana? Was he starting to show his age? Though his letter makes no mention of it, the 1880 census reveals that Caleb had a young son he had named John T. Moncrief. Indeed, Caleb must have thought of his father often.[49]

Letters came from Ireland and Germany, from family members who often had not seen their veteran since well before the war. Denis Hammafin, resident of County Kerry, Ireland, wrote to the asylum in 1891 rather desperate for information. He had written two years prior and gotten no response; now he asked if, "for god sake," the superintendent could tell him whether his son Timothy was alive or dead.[50] Two years later, the anxious father repeated his inquiry after another lapse in communication from the asylum. "I am sorely troubled and anxious about him, and would wish to hear as to how he is getting on," Hammafin begged.[51] Mary Carty wrote from Dublin in 1886 to ask about her husband, David, who had died in an attempt to escape the asylum. Mary's questions about the nature of her husband's condition went beyond the philosophical. She was entitled to a widow's pension, but she hadn't seen her husband in decades, and she had to rely on the doctors at the hospital to describe his body to her. "I would ask if his Insanity was caused by wounds received in late war or in active service," she wrote, "if there were gunshot or sword or bayonet wounds and where upon his person?"[52]

Parents and siblings often wrote to ask whether a veteran's condition could be improved with a different treatment or approach. Maria Sine wondered whether a surgery on her brother Henry Gibson's head, where he had been wounded, might help him to recover.[53] She wanted to be able to do something for him: "I wish i was able to do something for him or he was whare i could see him."[54] Franklin Hayes's siblings also wrote to the

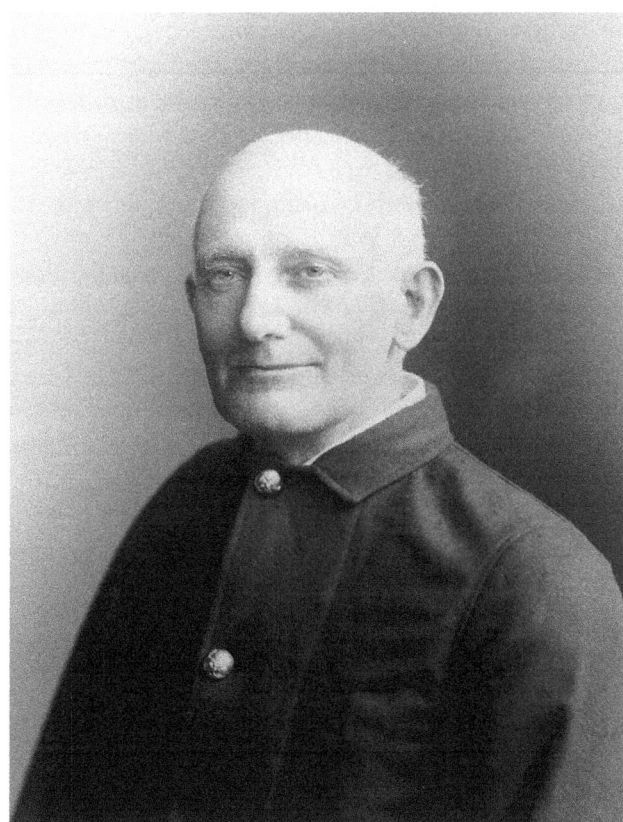

FIGURE 10. Franklin B. Hayes. Franklin B. Hayes case file, Record Group 418, St. Elizabeths Hospital, Case Records of Patients, 1855–1950, National Archives and Records Administration, Washington, DC.

superintendents of St. Elizabeths frequently, pushing doctors to provide the reasons for their brother's insanity. Franklin had lost an arm while serving the Eighth New Hampshire Infantry and had been committed to St. Elizabeths in 1870. It seemed that his family had never understood what had happened to him. Franklin's sister Lizzie wrote to Superintendent White in 1904, expressing her uncertainty about her brother's condition: "It occurs to me that there must be some *cause* for his present condition and that you have in all these years been unable to improve or ameliorate it."[55] It was possible he was a masturbator, she suggested, but how could that have caused such profound disability? Perhaps the war had been a catalyst, for, as Lizzie noted, "There is one thing certain—he was not born insane."[56]

The distance was particularly hard when families experienced times of trial at home. In January 1888, a father wrote to St. Elizabeths asking that a letter be read aloud to his son, Norton Bush, who had had been in the institution for many years. "My very dear Norton," he wrote, "your mother is no more an inhabitant of this earth."⁵⁷ In 1879, John Ira Rue's mother wrote to ask whether her son was ever lucid enough to receive news of his family. "If you think proper," she wrote, "tell him that his Brother Mark was lost on the Ocean going from Florida to NY."⁵⁸

Lizzie Wilson McReynolds's many letters to the superintendents of St. Elizabeths suggest that her brother John Wilson's condition was rarely far from her mind. In 1879, she quizzed W. W. Godding about John's condition. "Does he suffer mentally, and do you think he will ever recover his mind[?] Is there any hope[?] it is so hard to think he will never be sane again," she wrote. In another letter, McReynolds wanted even more detail: "What does he do and say, and talk about[?] does he say anything about home or any of his home folks[?] . . . Does he look old or care worn and do you make him work and does he ever read any or take an interest in anything[?]"⁵⁹ McReynolds, emotionally vulnerable following the death of her husband, was desperate to *know* her brother, whom she had not seen since she was a girl. Was he anything like the John she knew? Did he miss home? Was he comfortable, or did life in the asylum trouble him? She often asked the doctor to give her hope, but in reality, her own letters were her only hope. They were her sole opportunity to commune with her lost brother.

McReynolds struggled to reconcile her memories of John with his current reality. When she received a photograph taken of him in 1887, she was shocked at her brother's appearance: "Why, forty years seems to have passed over his head since [the last photograph]. What have you been doing to him[?] He looks like he has been abused and worked beyond the strength of [a] Human." There was no way he could look so worn and distressed, she reasoned: "My Brother was a very strong, healthy man and ought to be in his Prime, as he is only forty seven and his diseased mind ought not to make him look the Haggared creature as he appeared in that Picture."⁶⁰ McReynolds often wrote about her hopes to see her older brother, but she could never spare the money for the long trip to Washington. "I do want to see John again—It make[s] my Heart ache but I can't halp that I was not hardly grown when John went away."⁶¹

Letters also offered Lizzie McReynolds the chance to take care of John despite the hundreds of miles between them. Every Christmas, she sent John a box filled with candy, fruit, papers, and cigars. The Christmas box became central to her letters for weeks each year as she fretted about whether hospital staff allowed her brother free rein over his treats. "*Please* let him take it to his *own room*, where he can enjoy it at his leasure. If he wastes it, it is alright—it is his." She wanted to make sure that he had things that made him feel comforted and at home. "If you will tell me what John uses that the Home don't furnish, I will send it to him—such as tobacco and cigars—apples—fruits of different kinds."[62] It is particularly poignant that McReynolds had to ask the superintendent, who likely knew her brother better than she did at this point, what kinds of things he might like her to send.

Through her many questions and suggestions about John's condition, McReynolds contemplated the nature of her brother's mental illness. She struggled to understand what had caused it, and in letters written between the 1870s and the 1910s, she never indicated that she accepted the permanence of John's condition. The idea that he could live the rest of his life completely insensible was unfathomable. "It seems to me something could be done, John may live to be a very old man, and it is simply awfull that his mind would be blank all them years."[63] In one letter, written in 1900, she asked whether any doctor had examined John's head to see "if the pressure could not be lifted from his brains." Her theory of his illness stemmed from an incident that took place during the war: "In going up Lookout Mountain, in that bloody fight, John missed his footing and fell over a cliff and struck his head, knocking him senseless for a while."[64] After that, he was further stunned by the concussive blow of a nearby shell. How could it be possible that doctors could not somehow fix his skull, or relieve his brain? When science and technology could obscure the war's many lost arms and legs with prosthetics, it was galling that nothing could cure her brother. In this point, Lizzie McReynolds was not alone. Her father, David Wilson, admitted in an 1893 letter to the asylum that he also clung to the hope that John would someday improve: "I suppose it is follishness in me to think he will ever be well again but i cannot help it."[65]

As time went on, the hope that McReynolds asked the superintendents so often to provide began to fade, and she questioned whether John's disability had really been worth the sacrifice. In a 1909 letter, she dismissed the idea that his condition was part of a greater good. "How long do you think his weary worn life will last[?] It grieves me to think of his waisted lost life—and for *what*? The country. For him a great deal of good. If he had stayed at home what might he not have been today[?] Instead he is a wreck."[66] Just two years later, she seemed to lose her faith that her brother would ever improve enough to come home. Perhaps it would be better if he was dead. "My poor Brother will never be well again & it is nothing but a living death & continual sorrow to me," she wrote. "I would be glad if God would call him away so he would be at Rest." At least that way, she reasoned, she could be physically near her brother. "I could go to his Grave & It would seem I was near him."⁶⁷ She even went on to describe her final wishes for her brother: a good casket and a new blue suit befitting a Union soldier.

Lizzie McReynolds had been a child when her older brother went off to war, but in letter after letter, she described the emotional toll that her brother's mental illness had taken on her and her family. They might have escaped the ravages of the battlefield, but the pain of war trauma came to them anyway. Now, it seemed the most Lizzie McReynolds could hope for was to be reunited with her brother John in death.

In an 1864 letter to his sister, Daniel Folsom reflected on how he had ended up in the asylum at Utica. Mustering out of the Sixteenth New York was supposed to be the moment when his life returned to normal. Instead, the trials of the war just didn't seem to end. "I thought I had got through the hardest of my life when I got through solgerin," he lamented, "but if ever [I] got into a place where my life was a drug to me it is here."⁶⁸ Folsom was one of the lucky ones. Perhaps it wasn't the day he mustered out, but the day he walked out of Utica that marked the end of his war. Either way, Folsom's insight underlined a sentiment likely shared by a great many Union veterans, wounded in body and mind, for whom the Civil War did not end in the spring of 1865. But one wonders whether Folsom considered his sister's perspective—her war, in a sense, had not ended either.

Historians may never agree on the psychological impact of the Civil War. Whether a few, or some, or many, or all soldiers came home traumatized to some degree, and what we should call that trauma, will (and should) continue to spark debate. But the archive is not entirely silent. Asylum records hold the voices of soldiers and veterans, mothers and fathers, brothers and sisters, wives and children, all searching for ways to come to terms with the most invisible of war wounds. In their testimonies, these individuals almost always centered the war as the agent of change: a soldier left for the war as one man and came back as another. More importantly, soldiers and their loved ones described how that change set off chain reactions in their lives, altering their plans for the future and upending domestic harmony. But what seemed to pain many families most was the idea that mentally disabled soldiers were gone from their lives, but not from this life. They were trapped, far from home, living in a state somewhere between this world and the next. If some physically disabled veterans occupied a liminal state between hero and pauper, the mentally disabled occupied one between living and dead. The vacant chair remained empty, but so too did the grave.

EPILOGUE

Few would disagree that the Civil War wreaked havoc on bodies. We have long known that soldiers complained of sore feet, suffered from camp diseases, lived on poor rations, marched themselves into exhaustion, and, of course, had their flesh ripped and bones shattered. We can all conjure images of the disfigured bodies of soldiers photographed or painted at the direction of the Army Medical Department. So, too, can we envision the grotesque piles of discarded and disembodied limbs outside field hospitals. No pop-culture depiction and few historical examinations of the war would be complete without these images. The destruction of human bodies forms the bloody backdrop of this war.

The short-lived PBS drama *Mercy Street*, set in a Union hospital in Alexandria, Virginia, is a good example of the way our fascination with war's effects on the human body often plays out in popular culture. Set in a medical context, the show uses horrific injuries and diseases as plot devices, often quite powerfully. The series explores issues raised in recent scholarship, such as war trauma and health crises in contraband camps. However, wounded and sick soldiers exist within the show largely in a medical context. Suffering and gore lend dramatic intensity to the episodes, and wounds serve as problems for the main characters, all doctors and nurses, to solve. Having served their purpose, the wounded men fade into the background. Disabled soldiers and veterans often assume this role in Civil War scholarship: deployed to underscore the gravity of the contest or the commitment to the cause, but rarely placed at the center of the narrative. This is not to say that scholarship does not reveal these concepts. Rather, as I have endeavored to show, the experiences of such soldiers and veterans were about more than blood and honor.

The history of Civil War disability cannot be adequately understood when approached as medical problems to be solved, as abstract casualty numbers, or as red badges of courage. Disability profoundly changed the ways that soldiers existed in and interacted with their world. Soldiers praised as exemplars of Northern manhood were also mocked and segregated. They were stripped of the power to determine their own identity or to control their own bodies. As a result, soldiers struggled to maintain their balance on the fine line between patriotic manhood and dependency. Some believed that their wounds played a role in the Union victory. Others weren't so sure. Long after they had faded into the background of the main action, veterans continued to grapple with both the physical and social realities of wartime violence.

The history of Civil War disability continues to resonate today. As commercials for the Wounded Warrior Project attest, we again live in a time when amputees make up the central image of the war wounded. But less visible wounds also demand attention. Questions about the contours and ramifications of post-traumatic stress disorder and war trauma resurge anew after each war. They carry particular weight in the case of Sgt. Bowe Bergdahl, who faced court-martial for desertion while serving in Afghanistan. The experiences of the men court-martialed for seeking self-care are perhaps precedent for considering the extent to which the strain of war prompts a soldier like Bergdahl, with a history of mental illness, to leave his post. The wounds of soldiers like Joshua Lawrence Chamberlain are brought to mind by news that wounded veterans of Iraq and Afghanistan will be among the first to receive penis transplants in the United States. The Department of Veterans Affairs is also under increasing pressure to reverse its ban on paying for in vitro fertilization for former servicemen, largely in response to soldiers with line-of-duty genital trauma.[1] And like Abraham Griggs, veterans with bad reputations or dishonorable discharges continue to struggle to receive benefits. This is the case even when the behaviors that caused soldiers' "bad paper" stemmed from service-related traumas.[2]

In other ways unconnected with the military, disabled veterans' experiences foreshadow the situation modern-day disabled people face. Efforts are currently under way to place work requirements on Medicaid recipients in an effort to weed out the so-called "able-bodied." This development will undoubtedly mean that individuals with invisible or difficult-to-define ailments will again go unsupported.[3] The rollback of workers' compensation protections across the United States is also eerily reminiscent of Civil War veterans' struggles to secure pension payouts. Today's workers' compensation system particularly emphasizes rejecting claimants' requests by using legal and medical authorities' definitions of disability, definitions which are still linked to labor capacity.[4]

The Civil War was many things, but in a very practical sense it centered—as all wars do—on the destruction of the human body. Those who escaped the bullets and mortar shells still faced disease, exposure, and injury. Not every soldier became disabled, but nearly everyone who wore the blue Union uniform had a story about the things that war would do to a man. It was a central experience even for those who mustered out unmarked. Disability is a necessary by-product of war, and without coming to terms with that reality, we will never understand the full experience of this conflict, or any other.

NOTES

INTRODUCTION. Disability and the American Civil War

1. Doctorow, *March*, 2–70.
2. For examples of this scholarship, see Miller, *Empty Sleeves*; Nelson, *Ruin Nation*; Jordan, *Marching Home*; Downs, *Sick from Freedom*; Meier, *Nature's Civil War*; Clarke, *War Stories*; Devine, *Learning from the Wounded*; Sommerville, "Burden Too Heavy to Bear," 453–91; Sommerville, *Aberration of Mind*.
3. See, for example, Clarke, *War Stories*; Jordan, "Living Monuments."
4. See Skocpol, *Protecting Soldiers and Mothers*; Goldberg, *Citizens and Paupers*.
5. Belt, "Ballots for Bullets?," 441.
6. Greenberg, *Manifest Manhood*; Foote, *Gentlemen and the Roughs*.
7. Fraser and Gordon, "Genealogy of Dependency," 316. For a general discussion of the market revolution, see Wilentz, *Rise of American Democracy*; Sellers, *Market Revolution*; Howe, *What Hath God Wrought*. On antebellum disability, see Baynton, "Disability as a Justification for Inequality," in *New Disability History*, ed. Longmore and Umansky, 43–44; Nielsen, *Disability History of the United States*, 49–52.
8. Marten, "Nomads in Blue," in *Disabled Veterans in History*, ed. Gerber; Marten, *Sing Not War*; Jones, "Great Risk of Opium Eating."
9. Nielsen, *Disability History of the United States*, 87.
10. On overcoming rhetoric, see Rembis, "Athlete First," in *Disability and Passing*, ed. Brune and Wilson. On the supercrip, see Mitchell, "Beyond the Supercrip Syndrome," 18; Shapiro, *No Pity*, 12–40.
11. In recent years, the so-called dark turn has inspired much debate, and histories of disabled soldiers and veterans have been raised as an example of a "dark" interpretation of the Civil War experience. For examples, see Gallagher and Meier, "Coming to Terms," 487–508; Hess, "Where Do We Stand?," 371–403; Hsieh, "Go to Your Gawd Like a Soldier," 551–77.
12. Nielson, preface to *Disability History of the United States*, xiv.
13. Costa, "Changing Chronic Disease Rates," 119–37; Costa, "Mortality Declines"; Trulock, *In the Hands of Providence*, 174.
14. See Clarke, *War Stories*; Jordan, "Living Monuments"; Nelson, *Ruin Nation*.

CHAPTER 1. Gather the Invalids

1. Child, *History of the Fifth Regiment*, 154. Not only were its losses at Fredericksburg staggering, but at the end of the war, the Fifth New Hampshire also had the distinction of having the highest casualty rate of the entire Union army.

2. "Letter from a Member of the New Hampshire Fifth," *Farmer's Cabinet* (Amherst, NH), April 30, 1863.

3. "Letter from a Member of the New Hampshire Fifth," *Farmer's Cabinet* (Amherst, NH), April 30, 1863.

4. "Letter from a Member of the New Hampshire Fifth," *Farmer's Cabinet* (Amherst, NH), November 19, 1863.

5. Whites, *Civil War as a Crisis in Gender*.

6. For conflicting conceptions of manhood in the Union army, see Foote, *Gentlemen and the Roughs*.

7. See Rotundo, *American Manhood*, 233–35; Mitchell, *Vacant Chair*, 3–18; Linderman, *Embattled Courage*; Pettegrew, *Brutes in Suits*, 200–18. For a broader discussion of soldiers' motivation and reasons for enlistment, see McPherson, *What They Fought For, 1861–1865*; Hess, *Liberty, Virtue, and Progress*; Hess, *Union Soldier in Battle*; Prokopowicz, *All for the Regiment*; Gallagher, *Union War*.

8. See Baynton, "Disability as a Justification for Inequality," 43–44; Nielsen, *Disability History of the United States*, 49–52.

9. See Blackie, "Disability, Dependency, and the Family," in *Disability Histories*, ed. Rembis and Burch, 17–34.

10. See, for example, McCurry, *Masters of Small Worlds*; Hardesty, *Unfreedom*; Essah, *House Divided*; Jordan, *White Over Black*.

11. Fraser and Gordon, "Genealogy of Dependency," 316.

12. Clarke, *War Stories*, 152.

13. See Greenberg, *Manifest Manhood*; Foote, *Gentlemen and the Roughs*; Greenberg, *Honor and Slavery*; Johnson, *Sam Patch*; Gorn, *Manly Art*.

14. Frances Clarke calls this expectation "pluck." See Clarke, *War Stories*, 53, 72.

15. See for example, Emberton, "Only Murder Makes Men," 369–93; Cullen, "I's a Man Now," in *Divided Houses*, ed. Clinton and Silber, 76–91.

16. Cimbala, "Federal Manpower Needs," in *Scraping the Barrel*, ed. Marble, 7.

17. Humphreys, *Marrow of Tragedy*, 22.

18. Bartholow, *Manual of Instructions*, 210.

19. Bartholow, *Manual of Instructions*, 210.

20. "Letter from a Member of the N.H. Fifth," *Farmer's Cabinet* (Amherst, NH), April 5, 1863.

21. Humphreys, *Marrow of Tragedy*, 152–83.

22. General Orders No. 36, in United States War Department, *Official Records*, series 3, volume 2, page 9.(Subsequent citations from this source appear in this format: General Orders No. 36, *OR*, ser. 3, vol. 2, p. 9.) In addition, soldiers were sometimes contained at convalescent camps such as Camp Misery in Alexandria,

Virginia. These were known for poor discipline, poor hygiene, and supply shortages. See Adams, *Doctors in Blue*, 190; Schroeder-Lein, *Encyclopedia of Civil War Medicine*, 71–73.

23. Edwin Stanton, April 5, 1862, *OR*, ser. 3, vol. 2, p. 9.
24. Bartholow, *Manual of Instructions*, 216.
25. Humphreys, *Marrow of Tragedy*, 164.
26. Untitled article, *Bedford (PA) Gazette*, August 18, 1865.
27. Bellard, *Gone for a Soldier*, ed. Donald, 232–33.
28. "Letter from a Member of the N.H. Fifth," *Farmer's Cabinet* (Amherst, NH), July 5, 1863.
29. United States Sanitary Commission, *Hospital Transports*, 84.
30. See Humphreys, *Marrow of Tragedy*, 64; Schultz, *Women at the Front*.
31. John W. DeForest to Brig. Gen. James B. Fry, November 30, 1865, *OR*, ser. 3, vol. 5, p. 543.
32. See John W. DeForest to Brig. Gen. James B. Fry, November 30, 1865, *OR*, ser. 3, vol. 5, p. 543–44.
33. Cimbala, "Federal Manpower Needs," 7.
34. John W. DeForest to Brig. Gen. James B. Fry, November 30, 1865, *OR*, ser. 3, vol. 5, p. 544.
35. John W. DeForest to Brig. Gen. James B. Fry, November 30, 1865, *OR*, ser. 3, vol. 5, p. 544.
36. John W. DeForest to Brig. Gen. James B. Fry, November 30, 1865, *OR*, ser. 3, vol. 5, p. 543. DeForest served with the Twelfth Connecticut and in various capacities throughout the war. After being wounded, he was commissioned as a captain in the Invalid Corps. After the war, DeForest worked with the Freedmen's Bureau until 1867. He went on to become a writer, penning war-related books such as *Miss Ravenel's Conversion from Secession to Loyalty*. See Adam, *Unwritten War*, 165–67.
37. General Order 212, *OR*, ser. 3, vol. 3, p. 475. Surgeons and officers were also required to note on all discharge papers the soldier's condition upon leaving the service. This information was to indicate whether a man was fit for the Invalid Corps. The later General Order 173 amended General Order 105 to exclude commissioned officers from the requirement forbidding surgeons to discharge men still fit for Invalid Corps duty.
38. The pension system set in place for Revolutionary War veterans established precedent for understanding disability in terms of capacity for manual labor. Blackie, "Disability, Dependency, and the Family"; Daen, "Revolutionary War Invalid Pensions," 141.
39. Bartholow, *Manual of Instructions*, 250.
40. General Order 212, *OR*, ser. 3, vol. 3, pp. 475–78.
41. Barnes, *Medical and Surgical History*, part 3, volume 1, page 43. (Subsequent citations from this source appear in this format: Barnes, *MSHWR*, pt. 3, vol. 1, p. 43.) An article in the *Army and Navy Journal and Gazette* reported very different

findings in 1865, suggesting that gunshot wounds outweighed disease, but it's unclear where the statistics were drawn from, or whether they included the officers. See "Report of the Secretary of War," *Army and Navy Journal and Gazette*, July 1, 1865, in *Army and Navy Journal and Gazette, Vol. II 1864–1865*, 711.

42. As an example of how potential officers were evaluated, see Proceedings of the Board Established to Examine Officers of the Veteran Reserve Corps and Applicants for Appointment to the Corps, 1864–1865, Record of the Provost Marshal General's Bureau, Record Group 110, National Archives and Records Administration (hereafter cited as NARA), Washington, DC.

43. Cimbala, "Federal Manpower Needs," 11.

44. These numbers are based on the listing in the *Field Record of the Officers of the Veteran Reserve Corps*, published in 1865. The *MSHWR* indicates that there were 636, not 427, officers in the VRC, and that two-thirds of them were "subjects of gunshot wounds." This information seems to align with statistics from the *Field Record*. See John Moore, *MSHWR*, pt. 3, vol. 1, p. 43. A survey of one examining board's 1864 records makes it clear that wounded men were more likely to receive commissions. But it also seems as though men with chronic illnesses were less likely to seek a commission in the first place. Officers, it should be noted, had the option of resigning their commission rather than being required to transfer to the Invalid Corps. See Proceedings of the Board Established to Examine Officers of the Veteran Reserve Corps and Applicants for Appointment to the Corps, 1864–1865.

45. *Field Record*, 4.

46. *Field Record*, 20, 23. In 1866, while still serving in the corps, Lt. Louis Ahrens walked into a gun store in Washington, DC, asked to look at a pistol, and put the muzzle into his mouth and shot himself. No one could say why he had done it, but friends reported that he had been talking about suicide for a few days prior. "Suicide of an Army Officer at Washington," *Pittsfield (MA) Sun*, April 26, 1866. Ahrens's name is recorded elsewhere as Lewis Ahrene.

47. *Field Record*, 6.

48. James B. Fry to E. M. Stanton, November 17, 1863, *OR*, ser. 3, vol. 3, p. 1046.

49. James B. Fry to E. M. Stanton, November 17, 1863, *OR*, ser. 3, vol. 3, p. 1046.

50. Bartholow, *Manual of Instructions*, 212.

51. Suplick, "United States Invalid Corps / Veteran Reserve Corps," 48–49.

52. "Men Wanted for the Invalid Corps," *Farmer's Cabinet* (Amherst, NH), September 3, 1863.

53. "Miscellaneous. The Invalid Corps—What Its Duties Are," *National American* (Bel Air, MD), November 20, 1863.

54. Circular No. 14, *OR*, ser. 3, vol. 3, p. 225.

55. Cimbala, "Federal Manpower Needs," 8.

56. Donald, *Gone for a Soldier*, 236–78.

57. Cimbala, "Federal Manpower Needs," 16.

58. According to John W. DeForest, between its creation in April 1863 and September 30, 1865, the corps received 45,037 men by transfer from within the army, 5,275 enlisted men, and 3,032 reenlisted men. DeForest to Brig. Gen. James B. Fry, November 30, 1865, *OR*, ser. 3, vol. 5, p. 566.

59. "Letter from an Ex-Member of the N.H. Fifth Regiment," *Farmer's Cabinet* (Amherst, NH), November 9, 1863.

60. Walter Dunn to Emma Randolph, October 23, 1863, in *After Chancellorsville*, ed. Bailey and Cottom, 16.

61. Walter Dunn to Emma Randolph, December 7, 1863, in *After Chancellorsville*, ed. Bailey and Cottom, 22.

62. Walter Dunn to Emma Randolph, May 25, 1865, in *After Chancellorsville*, ed. Bailey and Cottom, 228.

63. DeForest to Brig. Gen. James B. Fry, November 30, 1865, *OR*, ser. 3, vol. 5, p. 552.

64. Soldiers' frustration at losing their old units is in line with what many historians argue about the importance of comradeship and community to morale. See, for example, McPherson, *For Cause and Comrades*; Linderman, *Embattled Courage*; Dunkelman, *Brothers One and All*.

65. "Why Are Not Colored Troops Received into the Veteran Reserve Corps?," *World* (New York, NY), January 5, 1865.

66. John W. DeForest to Brig. Gen. James B. Fry, November 30, 1865, *OR*, ser. 3, vol. 5, p. 549. See also Cimbala, "Federal Manpower Needs," 14; Pelka, ed., *Civil War Letters of Colonel Charles F. Johnson*, 14–15.

67. Beilein, "Guerrilla Shirt," 158.

68. In Pelka, ed., *Civil War Letters of Colonel Charles F. Johnson*, 238.

69. See Bourrier, *Measure of Manliness*; Frawley, *Invalidism and Identity*; Snyder, *Bachelors, Manhood, and the Novel*.

70. Sturgis, *Prisoners of War, 1861–1865*, 268–69. The name "Condemned Yanks" was also used by other Union soldiers. See Bellard, *Gone for a Soldier*, ed. Donald, 238.

71. In Cimbala, "Federal Manpower Needs," 13.

72. DeForest to Brig. Gen. James B. Fry, November 30, 1865, *OR*, ser. 3, vol. 5, p. 552.

73. Wilder, "Invalid Corps, Song & Chorus," Levy Sheet Music Collection, Box 088, Item 095, Johns Hopkins University Sheridan Libraries & University Museums, accessed on September 17, 2015, https://jscholarship.library.jhu.edu/handle/1774.2/23854. "Ticerdolerreou" refers to tic douloureux, or a facial tic. "Brown critters" most likely refers to lice.

74. "Why Are Not Colored Troops Received into the Veteran Reserve Corps?," *World* (New York, NY), January 5, 1865.

75. Suplick, "United States Invalid Corps / Veteran Reserve Corps," 69.

76. According to Slout, Buckley's Minstrels began in 1842 as the Congo Melodists. Slout, *Burnt Cork and Tambourines*, 55. For more on cultural depictions of black soldiers, see Fahs, *Imagined Civil War*, 162–94.

77. Mezurek, "De Bottom Rails on Top Now," in *Civil War Prisons II*, ed. Gray. Many thanks to Gray and Mezurek for sharing the manuscript with me.

78. Suplick, "United States Invalid Corps / Veteran Reserve Corps," 63.

79. Nelson deftly describes the importance of existing evidence of violence on black men's bodies in *Ruin Nation*, 172–75. For more on blackface minstrelsy, see Lott, *Love and Theft*.

80. See Boster, "Unfit for Ordinary Purposes," in *Disability Histories*, ed. Rembis and Burch, 201–17; Nielsen, *Disability History of the United States*, 56–66; Jefferson, "Enabled Courage," 1102–24.

81. Mezurek, "De Bottom Rails on Top Now," 9–10.

82. Mezurek, "De Bottom Rails on Top Now," 10.

CHAPTER 2. **Army of the Walking Sick**

1. The Forty-Sixth Article of War required a court-martial for any soldier caught sleeping at his post. US War Department, *The 1863 Laws of War* (Mechanicsburg: Stackpole Books, 2005), 14.

2. Ephraim Pelton court-martial, Court-Martial Case Files and Related Records, Record Group 153, Records of the Office of the Judge Advocate General (Army), 1792–2010, NARA, Washington, DC.

3. On the sometimes frustrating tension between the expectations of the citizen-soldier and expectations of the citizen, see Ramold, *Baring the Iron Hand*; Foote, *Gentleman and the Roughs*.

4. Moore, *MSHWR* pt. 3, vol. 1, pp. 24, 43.

5. The relationship between illness and disability is a point of debate for disability scholars. The social model of analysis argues that an inhospitable, ableist society creates incapacity, which would simply be difference without this barrier. Equating illness with disability, many argue, threatens to again yoke disability to the medical model of analysis. This interpretation considers disability a medical problem necessitating treatment and cure. I bring the two schools of thought together to argue that soldiers had physically and socially disabling ailments requiring treatment. Civil War–era Americans understood illness as disability because it prevented men from performing their military and, after the war, work duties. For more on the debate over illness and disability, see Shakespeare, *Disability Rights and Wrongs*; Shakespeare, *Disability Rights and Wrongs Revisited*; Shakespeare, "Debating Disability," 11–14; Wendell, "Unhealthy Disabled," 17–33; Johnstone, *Introduction to Disability Studies*; Albrecht, Seelman, and Bury, eds., *Handbook of Disability Studies*, 300–302; Barnes and Mercer, eds., *Exploring the Divide*.

6. See Lonn, *Desertion during the Civil War*; Weitz, *More Damning Than Slaughter*; Weitz, *Higher Duty*; Ramold, *Baring the Iron Hand*.

7. For example, Ella Lonn's classic work points to some of the physical difficulties of soldiering, such as insufficient supplies, poor food, and inadequate shoes,

warm clothes, or blankets, as potential causes for desertion. See Lonn, *Desertion during the Civil War*. Steven Ramold also discusses how health impacted insubordination. Ramold, *Baring the Iron Hand*, 184–92.

8. Meier, *Nature's Civil War*. Straggling (Article 41 of the 1863 Laws of War) was considered temporarily leaving the ranks with the intention of returning. Desertion (Article 20 of the 1863 Laws of War) was deemed leaving the ranks permanently. Steven Ramold offers a detailed exploration of the varying degrees of leaving the ranks without permission in *Baring the Iron Hand*, 220–63.

9. Meier, *Nature's Civil War*, 127. For more on the class- and gender-based tension between officers and enlisted men, see Foote, *Gentlemen and the Roughs*.

10. Meier, *Nature's Civil War*, 139–41.

11. See Lonn, *Desertion during the Civil War*, 157–58. Officers also believed that cowardly but able-bodied soldiers used aiding the sick and wounded as an excuse to leave the field. See Governor K. Warren to Seth Williams, January 15, 1864, *OR*, ser. 1, vol. 33, p. 379.

12. Lenker, *Civil War Memoir of Sgt. Christian Lenker*.

13. Abraham Lincoln to George B. McClellan, July 13, 1862, *OR*, ser. 1, vol. 11, pt. 3, p. 319.

14. General Order No. 61, *OR*, ser. 3, vol. 2, p. 112; General Order No. 65, *OR*, ser. 3, vol. 2, p. 146.

15. Maj. Gen. Joseph Hooker to Maj. Gen. Henry Halleck, January 30, 1863, *OR*, ser. 1, vol. 25, pp. 10–11; General Order No. 3, *OR*, ser. 1, vol. 25, pp. 11–12. See also Ramold, *Baring the Iron Hand*, 238–40.

16. John P. Hamilton to "Sister Mary," January 7, 1863, in *Brunswick and the Civil War*, ed. Rajoppi.

17. Ramold, *Baring the Iron Hand*; Meier, *Nature's Civil War*.

18. David Okes court-martial, Court-Martial Case Files and Related Records, Record Group 153, Records of the Office of the Judge Advocate General (Army), 1792–2010, NARA, Washington, DC. (Hereafter cited as David Okes court-martial.)

19. David Okes court-martial.

20. Alexander Cranston court-martial, Court-Martial Case Files and Related Records, Record Group 153, Records of the Office of the Judge Advocate General (Army), 1792–2010, NARA, Washington, DC.

21. Thomas A. Fenlan court-martial, Court-Martial Case Files and Related Records, Record Group 153, Records of the Office of the Judge Advocate General (Army), 1792–2010, NARA, Washington, DC.

22. Dennis Kelley court-martial, Court-Martial Case Files and Related Records, Record Group 153, Records of the Office of the Judge Advocate General (Army), 1792–2010, NARA, Washington, DC.

23. Elso Boelson court-martial, Court-Martial Case Files and Related Records, Record Group 153, Records of the Office of the Judge Advocate General (Army), 1792–2010, NARA, Washington, DC.

24. Thomas Jaegar court-martial, Court-Martial Case Files and Related Records, Record Group 153, Records of the Office of the Judge Advocate General (Army), 1792–2010, NARA, Washington, DC.

25. Henry Peers court-martial, Court-Martial Case Files and Related Records, Record Group 153, Records of the Office of the Judge Advocate General (Army), 1792–2010, NARA, Washington, DC.

26. Intestinal diseases had devastating effects on the Union army, killing over 46,000 men, and prompting a full 13 percent of all Union discharges. For reference, troop strength of the Union army between 1861 and 1865 was an estimated 2.6 million. For more on intestinal disease during the Civil War, see Kohl, "This Godforsaken Town," 118–19.

27. Wiley, *Life of Billy Yank*, 136. See also Meier, *Nature's Civil War*, 59–60.

28. Meier, *Nature's Civil War*, 7.

29. Clarke, *War Stories*, 72. See also Nelson, *Ruin Nation*, 185.

30. In McPherson, *For Cause and Comrades*, 26. Spelling in original.

31. Meier, *Nature's Civil War*, 133.

32. Moore, *MSHWR*, pt. 3, vol. 1, p. 836.

33. James McGrogan court-martial, Court-Martial Case Files and Related Records, Record Group 153, Records of the Office of the Judge Advocate General (Army), 1792–2010, NARA, Washington, DC.

34. In Wiley, *Life of Billy Yank*, 29.

35. Wiley, *Life of Billy Yank*, 86; Ramold, *Baring the Iron Hand*, 187.

36. Ramold, *Baring the Iron Hand*, 186–90; Lande, *Madness, Malingering, and Malfeasance*, 131–56.

37. For a brief description of how physicians sought to catch malingers, see Anderson and Anderson, "Nostalgia and Malingering," 161–65.

38. Moore, *MSHWR*, pt. 3, vol. 1, p. 836.

39. General Order No. 65, *OR*, ser. 3, Vol. 2, p. 146.

40. William Fuller served as an assistant surgeon in the First Michigan until 1863, when he was seriously wounded. He returned home on a disability discharge, finished medical school at the University of Michigan, and was subsequently commissioned as the head surgeon of his former unit. Castel, ed., "Many . . . Diseases Are . . . Feigned," 31.

41. See Meier, *Nature's Civil War*, 45–58.

42. Bartholow, *Manual of Instructions*, 118.

43. Bartholow, *Manual of Instructions*, 132.

44. Lande, *Madness, Malingering, and Malfeasance*, 149.

45. Strychnia and colchieum were commonly used nineteenth-century medicines.

46. Moore, *MSHWR*, pt. 3, vol. 1, pp. 836–37.

47. Moore, *MSHWR*, pt. 3, vol. 1, p. 126.

48. Moore, *MSHWR*, pt. 3, vol. 1, p. 706. Emphasis in original.

49. James McGrogan court-martial.

50. Peter Boyer court-martial, Court-Martial Case Files and Related Records, Record Group 153, Records of the Office of the Judge Advocate General (Army), 1792–2010, NARA, Washington, DC.

51. According to the *MSHWR*, 5,213 soldiers experienced nostalgia to a "morbid degree." Barnes, *MSHWR*, pt. 1, vol. 1, pp. 638–39.

52. For a detailed analysis of the medical response to nostalgia, see Clarke, "So Lonesome I Could Die," 253–82.

53. Clarke, "So Lonesome I Could Die," 256.

54. In Moore, *MSHWR*, pt. 3, vol. 1, p. 885.

55. Anderson and Anderson, "Nostalgia and Malingering," 156–66.

56. In Moore, *MSHWR*, pt. 3, vol. 1, p. 885.

57. In Moore, *MSHWR*, pt. 3, vol. 1, p. 885.

58. John O'Niel court-martial, Court-Martial Case Files and Related Records, Record Group 153, Records of the Office of the Judge Advocate General (Army), 1792–2010, NARA, Washington, DC. The spelling of Graaf's name here is as it appears in the case records, but it also appears in the Official Records as Graff. Similarly, the record features this spelling of O'Niel, while the unit roster of the First New York Volunteer Engineers uses O'Neill. The trial records contain no indication of O'Niel's punishment.

59. Bartholow, *Manual of Instructions*, 95.

60. Clarke, *War Stories*, 58.

61. Clarke, *War Stories*, 54. For more on the importance of how a soldier carried out the act of suffering, see Faust, *This Republic of Suffering*.

62. See, for example, Miller, *Empty Sleeves*; Downs, *Sick from Freedom*; Meier, *Nature's Civil War*, 8.

CHAPTER 3. The United States Government Is Entitled to All of You

1. Brinton, *Personal Memoirs*, 190. During his time as curator, Brinton had two assistants, William Moss and Brinton Stone. It is not clear which of the two men interacted with the young soldier—or whether the "assistant curator" was Brinton himself.

2. Brinton, *Personal Memoirs*, 190. Demanding one's limb back in person seems to have been rare. It was more common for surviving soldiers to write to the museum and request a photograph of their bones to keep as a memento. See Devine, *Learning from the Wounded*, 197.

3. See Blight, *Race and Reunion*; Jordan, *Marching Home*; Neff, *Honoring the Civil War Dead*; Faust, *This Republic of Suffering*; Janney, *Remembering the Civil War*; Janney, *Burying the Dead But Not the Past*; Nelson, *Ruin Nation*; Clarke, *War Stories*; Marten, *Sing Not War*; Marten, *America's Corporal*.

4. See, for example, Devine, *Learning from the Wounded*; Barbian, Sledzik, and Resznick, "Remains of War"; Connor and Rhode, "Shooting Soldiers"; Goler

and Rhode, "From Individual Trauma to National Policy," in *Disabled Veterans in History*, ed., Gerber, 163–84.

5. Devine, *Learning from the Wounded*, 211.

6. See, for example, Nielsen, *Disability History of the United States*; Longmore and Umansky, *New Disability History*; Wu, *Chang and Eng Reconnected*.

7. See Grob, *Mad among Us*; Tomes, *Art of Asylum-Keeping*; Whitaker, *Mad in America*. On the American medical community's treatment of black and Native bodies, see Washington, *Medical Apartheid*; Skloot, *Immortal Life of Henrietta Lacks*; Blakeley and Harrington, *Bones in the Basement*; Savitt, *Medicine and Slavery*; Gould, *Mismeasure of Man*; Fabian, *Skull Collectors*. The case of *Schloendorff v. Society of New York Hospital* provided the first critical testing of consent in 1914. Justice Benjamin Cardozo famously stated, "Every human being of adult years and in sound mind has a right to determine what shall be done with his own body." The term "informed consent" was born out of *Salgo v. Leland Stanford University Board of Trustees et al.* in 1957. This case concerned Martin Salgo, who was not notified of the risks of a surgery that resulted in paralysis. After *Salgo*, consent continued to evolve into the concept that we understand today. For more on the state of consent in nineteenth-century America and the development of informed consent in the mid-twentieth century, see Faden and Beauchamp, *History and Theory of Informed Consent*. On the theory of medical authority, see Foucault, *Birth of the Clinic*.

8. The idea that the soldier's body is government property is not entirely gone. Urban legends have made that claim for decades, asserting that soldiers have been court-martialed for allowing themselves to get sunburned. Jeff Schogol, "Can Troops Be Punished for Damaging Government Property if They Get a Sunburn?," *Stars and Stripes*, June 28, 2010.

9. Jordan, "Living Monuments," 121.

10. Herschbach, "Fragmentation and Reunion," 218.

11. See Nelson, *Ruin Nation*; Clarke, *War Stories*; Jordan, "Living Monuments"; Miller, *Empty Sleeves*; Kinder, *Paying with Their Bodies*.

12. For more on the broader history of American medicine, see Starr, *Social Transformation of American Medicine*; Rutkow, *Seeking the Cure*; Rosenberg, *Care of Strangers*.

13. Devine, *Learning from the Wounded*, 17.

14. Grace, *Army Surgeon's Manual*, 101.

15. Devine, *Learning from the Wounded*, 36.

16. Sappol, *Traffic in Dead Bodies*, 3–4.

17. See Sappol, *Traffic of Dead Bodies*. On the construction of medical epistemology in the nineteenth century, see Whooley, *Knowledge in the Time of Cholera*.

18. Sappol, *Traffic of Dead Bodies*, 122.

19. Stowe, *Uncle Tom's Cabin*, 256. Antebellum Americans saw great beauty in death and dying, and they articulated this beauty in literature. See Schantz, *Awaiting the Heavenly Country*, 97–126.

20. Sappol, *Traffic in Dead Bodies*, 4, 35.

21. Faust, *This Republic of Suffering*, 62.

22. Sappol, *Traffic in Dead Bodies*, 5. For the longer history of bodies used for dissection, see Richardson, *Death, Dissection, and the Destitute*. On the abundance of bodies available during the Civil War, see Devine, *Learning from the Wounded*, 53–94.

23. Many thanks to Michael Rhode for his help in making sense of Circular No. 2.

24. Devine, *Learning from the Wounded*, 34.

25. Richardson, *Death, Dissection, and the Destitute*.

26. Brinton, *Personal Memoirs*, 180–81. Brinton and others often referred to the museum as a "cabinet." This old term had originally been used more or less interchangeably with "museum," but it came to specifically refer to a museum that held fantastic or rare items, particularly anatomical ones. See Crane, "Curious Cabinets and Imaginary Museums," in *Museums and Memory*, ed. Crane.

27. It was difficult for Brinton to procure such large quantities of alcohol, especially when it was carefully monitored so that troops did not overindulge. The surgeon general worked out a deal with Secretary of War Edwin Stanton that the museum would receive all liquor confiscated from soldiers within Washington, DC. Brinton was often frustrated to find that his barrels of whiskey were considerably lighter after their train journey from Washington to the front lines. Unsurprisingly, he discovered that soldiers were tapping into his barrels on the train and "sampling" the brew. One hopes that no one attempted this stunt on the return trip to Washington, when the barrels contained more than just whiskey. Brinton, *Personal Memoirs*, 191–92.

28. Brinton, *Personal Memoirs*, 186.

29. Brinton, *Personal Memoirs*, 187.

30. Herschbach, "Fragmentation and Reunion," 215–30.

31. Billings, *Medical Museums*, 27.

32. Harrison, *Dark Trophies*, 62.

33. Brinton, *Personal Memoirs*, 220.

34. For more, see Sappol, *Traffic in Dead Bodies*, 274–309.

35. Devine, *Learning from the Wounded*, 183.

36. Dan Sickles visited his leg every year on the anniversary of its amputation. Herschbach, "Fragmentation and Reunion," 241.

37. Billings, *Medical Museums*, 26.

38. Ames, *Ten Years in Washington*, 483. It is not clear how the wound was sustained.

39. Ames, *Ten Years in Washington*, 484. The same description is included in Bagger, "Army Medical Museum in Washington," *Appleton's Journal*, March 1, 1873. Mary Clemmer Ames might have consulted Bagger's work before writing her own very similar report of the museum.

40. Barnes, *MSHWR*, pt. 1, vol. 2, p. 261.

41. Barnes, *MSHWR*, pt. 1, vol. 2, p. 221.

42. For more on craniometry and similarly racist pseudosciences, see Gould, *Mismeasure of Man*; Fabian, *Skull Collectors*.

43. Kyle, "Army Medical Library and Museum," *Godey's Magazine*, June 1898, 416.

44. Fabian, *Skull Collectors*; see also Redman, *Bone Rooms*.

45. Kyle, "Army Medical Museum," 413.

46. In the summer of 1863, the Fifty-Fourth Massachusetts carried out a doomed assault on Fort Wagner in South Carolina. The regiment's white commander, Col. Robert Gould Shaw, was killed, along with many of his black soldiers. When enemy forces interred the dead, they purposely buried Shaw with his men. When comrades requested Shaw's body back, a Confederate officer replied that the Rebels had "buried him with his niggers." See Neff, *Honoring the Civil War Dead*, 62.

47. The bones of both soldiers and Natives were used in attempts to measure human bodies, further blurring the lines of supposed difference between the two collections. See Fabian, *Skull Collectors*, 165–203.

48. Brinton, *Personal Memoirs*, 190–91.

49. Brinton, *Personal Memoirs*, 191.

50. Edward Donnelly court of inquiry, Court-Martial Case Files and Related Records, Record Group 153, Records of the Office of the Judge Advocate General (Army), 1792–2010, NARA, Washington, DC. (Hereafter cited as Edward Donnelly court of inquiry.) Donnelly's case is also described in Lowry and Welsh, *Tarnished Scalpels*.

51. Edward Donnelly court of inquiry.

52. For a description of Barnum's American Museum, see Adams, *E Pluribus Barnum*, 75–115.

53. Edward Donnelly court of inquiry.

54. Edward Donnelly court of inquiry. Donnelly practiced medicine until his death in 1891. *Philadelphia College of Pharmacy Alumni Report*, vol. 28, p. 200.

55. See Nelson, *Ruin Nation*, 157, 228–32. Guerrillas were particularly notorious for taking Union scalps, which they often hung from the bridles of their horses. See Beilein, "Guerrilla Shirt," 176–79; Fellman, *Inside War*, 188–89.

56. Harrison, *Dark Trophies*, 100–102.

57. Edward Donnelly court of inquiry.

58. Edward Donnelly court of inquiry.

59. Claim for Widow's Pension with Minor Children, Sarah Anderson Pension File, certificate 121, 303, Record Group 15, Case Files of Approved Pension Applications of Widows and Others Who Served Mainly in the Civil War and the War With Spain, 1861–1934, NARA, Washington, DC; George Potts court-martial, Court-Martial Case Files and Related Records, Record Group 153, Records of the Office of the Judge Advocate General (Army), 1792–2010, NARA, Washington, DC. (Hereafter cited as George Potts court-martial.)

60. George Potts court-martial.

61. George Potts court-martial; Lowry and Welsh, *Tarnished Scalpels*, 71–72. Anderson's head was reunited with the rest of his body, and he was buried near Fort Harrison, Virginia. The graveyard is now a gravel quarry.

62. For instance, during a 1989 construction project on the building that had once been the Medical College of Georgia, workers unearthed nearly ten thousand human bones and skulls beneath the basement floor. According to studies of the remains, many dated back 1835, and 75 percent of them were African American. See Washington, *Medical Apartheid*, 120.

63. Cooper Owens, *Medical Bondage*; Fett, *Working Cures*, 151. Sims operated on nonconsenting slave men and women. In 1845, he removed an osteosarcoma from the jaw of a slave named Sam, whom medical students held down in the operating chair during the procedure. Sims later boasted of how useful the surgery was, even when the patient was unwilling. Washington, *Medical Apartheid*, 101–3.

64. During her tour of the United States in the mid-1830s, English writer Harriet Martineau observed that in Baltimore, the bodies of blacks were almost exclusively taken for dissection. She explained the practice as follows: "[The] whites do not like it and the coloured people cannot resist." See Humphreys, *Intensely Human*, 100.

65. See Fry, *Night Riders in Black Folk History*, 170–230. For more on night doctors, black body snatching, and medical experimentation on slaves and free blacks, see Washington, *Medical Apartheid*; Skloot, *Immortal Life of Henrietta Lacks*; Blakeley and Harrington, *Bones in the Basement*; Savitt, *Medicine and Slavery*.

66. George Potts court-martial.

67. Glatthaar, *Forged in Battle*, 192.

68. Potts was not the only doctor who ran into trouble for maltreating the body of a black soldier. Charles Briggs, the surgeon of the famed Fifty-Fourth Massachusetts, was called to investigate a possible case of bestiality between a private and mare. Finding some circumstantial evidence, Briggs had Pvt. James Riley held to a bed while he forcibly circumcised him, then cauterized his penis with a hot iron. Robert Gould Shaw, commander of the Fifty-Fourth, was appalled, but the incident resulted in no charges. Briggs lived a long, successful life, while Private Riley was killed at James Island, South Carolina, with a great many others of his storied unit. Lowry and Welsh, *Tarnished Scalpels*, 77–78.

69. Devine, *Learning from the Wounded*, 180.

70. Ames, *Ten Years in Washington*, 477.

71. "Ghastly Relics," *Weekly Telegraph* (Macon, GA) from the *Washington Star* (Washington, DC), October 6, 1885.

72. Woodward, "Army Medical Museum at Washington," *Lippincott's Magazine of Literature, Science and Education*, March 1877, 235.

73. Henry Van Ness Boynton (H. V. N. B.), "Letter from Washington," *Cincinnati Gazette*, March 9, 1866. Boynton, the lieutenant colonel of the Thirty-Fifth

Ohio, had been severely wounded at Chickamauga. He was awarded a medal of honor for his actions in that battle. For background on Boynton, see Summers, *Press Gang*; Smith, *Chickamauga Memorial*.

CHAPTER 4. The Disabled Lion of Union

Portions of this chapter were previously published in the *Journal of the Civil War Era* and the *New York Times*. See Handley-Cousins, "'Wrestling at the Gates of Death': Joshua Lawrence Chamberlain and Nonvisible Disability in the Civil War North," *Journal of the Civil War Era* 6 (June 2016): 220–42; "Wounded Lion of Union," *New York Times Disunion*, July 5, 2013.

1. Joshua Lawrence Chamberlain (hereafter referred to as JLC), "Charge at Fort Hell," William Henry Noble Papers, Rubenstein Library, Duke University, Durham, NC, 2.

2. JLC, "Charge at Fort Hell," 12–13.

3. JLC to Sarah "Sae" Chamberlain Farrington, January 29, 1882, JLC Papers, University of Maine, Orono Special Collections, copy in JLC Collection, Pejepscot Historical Society, Brunswick, ME.

4. JLC, "Charge at Fort Hell," 14.

5. JLC, "Charge at Fort Hell," 14.5.

6. JLC, "Charge at Fort Hell," 17.

7. Barnes, *MSHWR*, pt. 2, vol. 2, p. 363.

8. JLC to Sarah "Sae" Chamberlain Farrington, January 20, 1914, JLC Papers, University of Maine, Orono Special Collections, copy in JLC Collection, Pejepscot Historical Society.

9. JLC to Frances "Fanny" Caroline Adams Chamberlain, January 23, 1894, JLC Collection, Bowdoin College Special Collections, Brunswick, ME.

10. Surgeon's Certificate, 1893, JLC Military Pension Records, certificate 96, 956, Pension Application Files Based Upon Service in the Civil War and Spanish American War, Record Group 15, Records of the Veterans Administration, 1783–1985, NARA, Washington, DC.

11. Demographer and historian J. David Hacker argues that the estimated death toll of the Civil War is higher than has long been thought. The higher number owes in part to men like Chamberlain, men who died because of war wounds but not during the war years. See Hacker, "Census Based Count of the Civil War Dead," 307–48.

12. Baynton, "Disability as a Justification for Inequality," 52.

13. Paul Cimbala indicates the importance of this middle ground in his introduction to *Veterans North and South*. For interpretations of veterans, see Clarke, *War Stories*; Jordan, *Marching Home*; Casey, *New Men*; Marten, *Sing Not War*; Marten, *America's Corporal*; Nelson, *Ruin Nation*; Padilla, "Army of 'Cripples'"; Gannon, *Won Cause*. For examples of the debate over veterans' postwar lives, see Gallagher and Meier, "Coming to Terms"; Hess, "Where Do We Stand?"; Hsieh, "Go to Your Gawd Like a Soldier."

14. Skocpol, *Protecting Soldiers and Mothers*, 104; Barnes, *MSHWR*, pt. 3, vol. 2, p. 877. This number does not account for those whose wounds were missed by record keepers, those with psychological ailments, or the significant numbers of men who were disabled by wartime illnesses. In his study of the Civil War South, Brian Craig Miller articulates why it is critical to understand the role of amputation and amputees. See Miller, *Empty Sleeves*.

15. Davis, "Invisible Disability," 205. Tobin Siebers also discusses the ways in which able-bodiedness is itself "invisible because it is the norm." For disability to be perceived as real, it must be clearly apparent that a person is not able-bodied. Thus, Siebers argues, visibly disabled people face greater discrimination. This was not always the case in the Civil War era, as war wounds were associated with honor and heroism. See Siebers, *Disability Theory*, 102–3.

16. Clarke, *War Stories*, 151.

17. See Nelson, *Ruin Nation*; Marten, *Sing Not War*; Clarke, *War Stories*; Miller, *Empty Sleeves*, 102–4. Some men preferred it this way. Brian Craig Miller conveys the story of Confederate veteran Charles Rainwater, who was thankful that no one could see the "reminder of the war" on his body. Miller, *Empty Sleeves*, 122.

18. Rembis, "Athlete First," 113.

19. Another useful way of looking at this subject is through the "supercrip" trope, an overcoming narrative in which disabled people would be pitiable but for their extraordinary actions or abilities. Many Civil War veterans who enjoyed happy or successful postwar lives are described in terms of the supercrip. See Mitchell, "Beyond the Supercrip Syndrome," 18; Shapiro, *No Pity*, 12–40. For more on how Chamberlain has become mythologized, and the role his wound played in that process, see Pullen, *Joshua Chamberlain*, 172.

20. I intentionally use the term *cripple* here to evoke nineteenth-century terminology. Rembis, "Athlete First," 116. The concept of *double consciousness* was also articulated in Du Bois, *Souls of Black Folk*.

21. JLC, "Through Blood and Fire at Gettysburg," *Hearst's Magazine*, January 1913, 909.

22. For examples, see JLC, *The Passing of the Armies* (New York: G. P. Putnam's Sons, 1915), 34, 271, 308–10, 316. Many of these passages also invoke very dark imagery along with the language of sacrifice, bravery, and patriotism. For a discussion of the importance of sentimental writing to Civil War–era Americans, see Clarke, *War Stories*. Wayne Hsieh notes that many veterans felt a "nostalgia for war," and he traces the ways that many historians have highlighted it. See Hsieh, "Go to Your Gawd Like a Soldier," 553.

23. JLC, "Charge at Fort Hell," 2.

24. Sarah D. B. Chamberlain to JLC, January 1, 1865, Chamberlain-Adams Collection, Schlesinger Library, Radcliffe College, Cambridge, MA, copy in JLC Collection, Pejepscot Historical Society.

25. JLC to Sarah D. B. Chamberlain, undated, JLC Collection, Bowdoin College Special Collections. The "dear ones" Chamberlain referred to were his wife, Frances Caroline Adams Chamberlain, and small children.

26. JLC to Joshua Chamberlain Jr., February 20, 1865, JLC Collection, Bowdoin College Special Collections.

27. Herr, "Privates Were Shot," in *Years of Change and Suffering*, ed. Schmidt and Hasegawa, 98.

28. Herr, "Privates Were Shot," 96.

29. Herr, "Privates Were Shot," 89, 96.

30. Surgeon's Certificate, 1893, JLC Military Pension Records, certificate 96, 956.

31. Trulock, *In the Hands of Providence*, 219; JLC to John Chamberlain Jr., December 19, 1864, JLC Collection, Bowdoin College Special Collections.

32. Rev. George Adams Diary, May 22, 1865, First Parish Church, Brunswick, ME. I am indebted to First Parish Church archivist Mildred Jones for graciously granting me access to the reverend's diaries.

33. Interview of Catherine T. Smith by Isabel Whittier, January 16, 1961, JLC Collection, Pejepscot Historical Society. This chair is on display at the Chamberlain House in Brunswick, Maine.

34. Jane "Jenny" Abbott to JLC, May 20, 1872, Chamberlain-Adams Collection, Schlesinger Library, Radcliffe College, Cambridge, MA.

35. Jane "Jenny" Abbott to JLC, undated [1868], Chamberlain-Adams Collection. It seems a reasonable interpretation of Jenny's intimate letters to Chamberlain that she had feelings for him, but we have no evidence that he reciprocated. See Smith, *Fanny & Joshua.*

36. JLC to Frances "Fanny" Caroline Adams Chamberlain, summer 1852, quoted in Smith, *Fanny & Joshua*, 40. See also Pullen, *Joshua Chamberlain*, 111–12. On the Chamberlain marriage, see also Jennifer Lund Smith, "Reconstruction of 'Home': The Civil War and the Marriage of Lawrence and Fanny Chamberlain," in *Intimate Strategies of the Civil War*, ed. Bleser and Gordon.

37. JLC to Fanny Chamberlain, July 24, 1863, original letter in private collection, quoted in Smith, *Fanny & Joshua*, 145. Not long after this letter was written, the "unsoundness of mind" to which Chamberlain referred worsened, and he was granted a furlough to recover from nervous prostration.

38. When writing *In the Hands of Providence*, Alice Trulock consulted urologist George Files. In a letter to Trulock, Dr. Files wrote, "It would seem to me that with his bouts of wound pain along with urinary frequency, dysuria, and a tender fistula bed, there were more than enough distracting factors to dampen any erotic desires." This is not to suggest that disabled people are incapable of full and satisfying sexual lives, but it seems any sexual relationship Fanny and Joshua shared was likely much altered. Dr. Files's notes are in the JLC Medical File, Pejepscot Historical Society. See also Harmon and McAllister, "Lion of the Union"; McAllister, "Fire, Blood, and the Lion of the Union"; Pullen, *Joshua Chamberlain*, 111–12.

39. Trulock, *In the Hands of Providence*, 338–41.

40. JLC to Frances "Fanny" Caroline Adams Chamberlain, November 20, 1868, Frost Family Papers, Yale University Library, copy in JLC Collection, Pejepscot Historical Society.

41. JLC to Frances "Fanny" Caroline Adams Chamberlain, November 20, 1868, Frost Family Papers, Yale University Library, copy in Joshua Lawrence Chamberlain Collection, Pejepscot Historical Society.

42. Smith, *Chickamauga Memorial*, 13–15.

43. Charles F. Johnson to Mary Johnson, April 7, 1864, in *Civil War Letters of Colonel Charles F. Johnson*, ed. Pelka, 225. Spelling in original.

44. Nelson, *Ruin Nation*, 197–99.

45. See Miller, *Empty Sleeves*, 91–115; Nelson, *Ruin Nation*, 197–200.

46. Miller, *Empty Sleeves*, 102.

47. Smith, *Fanny & Joshua*, 196.

48. Chamberlain also contracted malaria while in the army, and this might have compounded his ill health. According to Dora L. Costa, malaria led to increased chronic disease and decreased ability to work among affected Union veterans late in their lives. See Costa, "Changing Chronic Disease Rates," 119–37; Costa, "Mortality Declines." Chamberlain contracted a "malarial fever" in 1862. Trulock, *In the Hands of Providence*, 174.

49. Dr. Joseph H. Warren to JLC, March 2, 1883, Frost Family Papers, Yale University Library, copy in JLC Collection, Pejepscot Historical Society.

50. "Gen. J. L. Chamberlain's Wound," *New York Times*, March 18, 1883.

51. John Bigelow to JLC, April 27, 1883, Correspondence, Joshua Lawrence Chamberlain, 1828–1914, Maine Historical Society, Portland, ME, copy in JLC Collection, Pejepscot Historical Society.

52. Frances "Fanny" Caroline Adams Chamberlain to JLC, April 21, 1883, original in private collection, copy in the Alice Rains Trulock Papers, Pejepscot Historical Society.

53. *Portland (ME) Transcript*, April 25, 1883, clipping in JLC Collection, Pejepscot Historical Society. The article has no listed author, and it gives no indication of who provided the newspaper with information about the wound or the surgery.

54. Nelson, *Ruin Nation*, 160–227; Clarke, *War Stories*, 144–74.

55. The *Portland (ME) Transcript*, April 25, 1883, clipping in JLC Collection, Pejepscot Historical Society.

56. Holmes, *Soundings from the Atlantic*, 282–327.

57. Holmes, *Soundings from the Atlantic*, 317.

58. For more on Civil War sentimental literature and disabled Union veterans, see Clarke, *War Stories*.

59. "The Veteran," *Harper's Weekly*, January 5, 1867.

60. David Barker, "The Empty Sleeve," in *Rebellion Record*, ed. Moore, 47.

61. *New York Times*, July 27, 1883, clipping in the JLC Collection, Pejepscot Historical Society.

62. JLC to Sarah "Sae" Chamberlain Farrington, July 3, 1883, JLC Papers, Library of Congress, copy in JLC Collection, Pejepscot Historical Society. Emphasis in original.

Notes to Chapter Four

63. Affidavit of Fitz John Porter, JLC Military Pension Records, certificate 96, 956, Pension Application Files Based Upon Service in the Civil War and Spanish American War, Record Group 15, Records of the Veterans Administration, 1783–1985, NARA, Washington, DC.

64. "Medical Referee's Instructions to the Examining Physician," March 1893, JLC Military Pension Records, certificate 96, 956. For more on the difficulty of getting a pension with a nonvisible wound, see Blanck and Millender, "Before Disability Civil Rights," 5; Logue and Blanck, *Race, Ethnicity and Disability*, 73–78.

65. Siebers, *Disability Theory*, 102–3.

66. JLC to Pension Bureau, February 6, 1893, JLC Military Pension Record, certificate 96, 956.

67. Surgeon's Certificate, 1893, JLC Military Pension Record, certificate 96, 956.

68. Untitled document, September 1893, JLC Military Pension Record, certificate 96, 956.

69. Eliot, *President Eliot's Speech*, 3–4.

70. See Logue and Blanck, *Race, Ethnicity and Disability*, 77.

71. Photograph No. 93, *Recovery after a Penetrating Gunshot Wound of the Abdomen, with Perforation of the Left Ilium*, Surgical Photographs, 1860s–1880s, OHA 82, Otis Historical Archives, National Museum of Health and Medicine (NMHM), Silver Spring, MD; "Death of General Barnum," *New York Tribune*, February 2, 1892, Henry A. Barnum Collection, Onondaga Historical Association, Syracuse, NY.

72. Photograph No. 93, *Recovery after a Penetrating Gunshot Wound*.

73. Henry A. Barnum Military Pension Records, certificate 78, 753, Pension Application Files Based Upon Service in the Civil War and Spanish American War, Record Group 15, Records of the Veterans Administration, 1783–1985, NARA, Washington, DC.

74. Henry A. Barnum to Colonel Lockwood, January 6, 1888, Henry A. Barnum Military Pension Records, certificate 78, 753.

75. Henry A. Barnum Collection, Onondaga Historical Association. It is not clear when, why, or by whom these pictures were taken, but they don't match the style of those taken for the Army Medical Museum and the *MSHWR*. Nor do copies of these photographs exist at the Otis Historical Archives, leading me to conclude they were made privately.

76. The *Syracuse Courier* from the *Albany (NY) Journal*, July 21, 1881, clipping in the Henry A. Barnum Collection, Onondaga Historical Association.

77. "In Honor of Gen. Barnum," *New York Times*, August 8, 1889.

78. Trulock, *In the Hands of Providence*, 369; Pullen, *Joshua Chamberlain*, 153. In Pullen's estimation, Chamberlain was cash poor from bad investments and business failures, but he still owned property. Without added income, he would have had to start selling off assets.

79. Trulock, *In the Hands of Providence*, 369.

80. JLC to Sarah "Sae" Chamberlain Farrington, January 20, 1914, JLC Collection, University of Maine, Orono Special Collections, copy in JLC Collection, Pejepscot Historical Society.

CHAPTER 5. Man or Mercenary

Portions of this chapter were previously published in the *New York Times* and *Nursing Clio*. Please see Handley-Cousins, "PTSD and the Civil War," *New York Times*, August 13, 2014; "Disability, Responsibility, and the Veteran Pension Paradox," *Nursing Clio*, January 30, 2014.

1. For instance, not including pocket vetoes, Chester A. Arthur and James Buchanan vetoed only four bills during their tenure, while Abraham Lincoln and James K. Polk only vetoed two. "Vetoes: Summary of Bills Vetoed, 1789–present," United States Senate website, https://www.senate.gov/reference/Legislation/Vetoes/vetoCounts.htm.
2. "Veto of the Bill Granting a Pension to Abraham P. Griggs," *Public Papers of Grover Cleveland*, 228. Cleveland read many of the pension files himself, but in some cases he asked Commissioner of Pensions John C. Black to offer recommendations on the bills.
3. Surgeon's Certificate, Abraham P. Griggs, May 24, 1885, Abraham P. Griggs Pension File, certificate number 688, 275, Pension Application Files Based Upon Service in the Civil War and Spanish American War, Record Group 15, Records of the Veterans Administration, 1783–1985, NARA, Washington, DC.
4. Skocpol, *Protecting Soldiers and Mothers*, 109, 111–18.
5. Marten, *America's Corporal*, 99.
6. Jordan, *Marching Home*, 11.
7. Skocpol, *Protecting Soldiers and Mothers*, 109.
8. "Charged with Pension Fraud," *Daily Inter Ocean* (Chicago, IL), January 16, 1894.
9. "Charged with Pension Fraud," *Daily Inter Ocean* (Chicago, IL), January 16, 1894.
10. Marten, *Sing Not War*, 218. See also Marten, *America's Corporal*, 92–130.
11. Skocpol, *Protecting Soldiers and Mothers*, 143–44. Further, when investigations to review unworthy pensions were launched in 1873 and again between 1876 and 1879, the number of cases dropped for being "fraudulent" amounted to only 0.5 percent of the total pensions on the rolls.
12. See Smith, *Enemy Within*; Marten, *Sing Not War*, 213–23.
13. "A Pension Fraud," *Jackson (MI) Citizen*, January 8, 1895; "Charged with Pension Fraud," *Kansas City (MO) Times*, November 14, 1895.
14. "Deserted Twice and Wants a Pension," *Daily Herald* (Grand Forks, ND), August 18, 1890.
15. Untitled article, *Daily Register* (Rockford, IL), August 27, 1889.
16. Bartholow, *Manual of Instructions*, 94–95.

17. In McPherson, *For Cause and Comrades*, 9. See also Casey, "Marked by War," 123–51; Grant, "Citizen-Soldiers, Disabled Veterans, and Confederate Nationalism," 233–54; Pettegrew, *Brutes in Suits*, 197–268.

18. "No Difference Between a Veteran and a Bummer," *New York Herald*, August 25, 1889.

19. Wiley, *Life of Billy Yank*, 48–49.

20. "Exactly in Point," *Portland Oregonian*, February 25, 1887.

21. Summers, *Rum, Romanism, & Rebellion*, 49.

22. "The Volunteer and the Mercenary," *St. Louis Republic*, December 8, 1888.

23. For a breakdown of the numbers of veterans pensioned by decade, see Skocpol, *Protecting Soldiers and Mothers*, 109.

24. "Exactly in Point," *Portland Oregonian*, February 25, 1887.

25. "A Word for Gen. Tannatt," *Portland Oregonian*, March 8, 1887.

26. "Rich Men Accepting Alms," *Portland Oregonian*, October 23, 1889.

27. "The Southern Soldier," *New York Herald*, July 7, 1889. Spelling in original.

28. Miller, *Empty Sleeves*, 160–63, 172. For more on the South's support for disabled veterans, see Hasegawa, *Mending Broken Soldiers*.

29. Quoted in Miller, *Empty Sleeves*, 162.

30. Miller, *Empty Sleeves*, 161.

31. For an excellent, in-depth discussion of pensions in the former Confederacy, see Miller, *Empty Sleeves*, 141–72.

32. Costa and Kahn, *Heroes & Cowards*, 169. Costa and Kahn suggest that while these laws were not heavily enforced, their presence was enough to encourage many dishonorably discharged soldiers to leave their hometowns.

33. "Pensioning Deserters," *Times-Picayune* (New Orleans, LA), October 15, 1890.

34. "The Malingerers of 1863 and 1897," *New York Sun*, December 29, 1897.

35. "Malingerers of 1863 and 1897," *New York Sun*, December 29, 1897.

36. Skocpol, *Protecting Soldiers and Mothers*, 108, 588. Skocpol writes, "Interestingly, the 28 percent rejection rate is considerably lower than the rejection rate of about 28 percent for the entire period from 1861–1888. Presumably, applications in the period during and right after the Civil War were more likely to be corroborated by hard evidence of death or disability." *Protecting Soldiers and Mothers*, 588.

37. "Word for Gen. Tannatt," *Portland Oregonian*, March 8, 1887.

38. Padilla, "Army of 'Cripples,'" 102. See also Logue and Blanck, *Race, Ethnicity and Disability*, 17. For more on manhood and class in the North, see Foote, *Gentlemen and the Roughs*; Rotundo, *American Manhood*; Greenberg, *Manifest Manhood*.

39. Roosevelt, *Strenuous Life*.

40. On football, see Edwards, *New Spirits*, 121–24; and Pettegrew, *Brutes in Suits*, 128–79. On changes in men's clothing, see Hill, *American Menswear*, 84–88. For more on late nineteenth-century masculinity, see Kasson, *Houdini, Tarzan, and The Perfect Man*; Bederman, *Manliness & Civilization*; Hoganson, *Fighting for American Manhood*.

41. This practice was in keeping with the policy for disabled veterans of earlier wars. See Blackie, "Disability, Dependency, and the Family," 18; Daen, "Revolutionary War Invalid Pensions," 141.

42. For more on labor and disabled veterans, see Padilla, "Army of 'Cripples,'" 67–108; Marten, *Sing Not War*, 236–40. An 1874 report noted that work requiring "skill and education" should also be included under the umbrella of "manual labor," but this determination did not seem to make much difference in disability ratings. Costa, *Evolution of Retirement*, 198–99.

43. Padilla, "Army of 'Cripples,'" 99.

44. See Padilla, "Army of 'Cripples'"; Miller, *Empty Sleeves*; Marten, *Sing Not War*, 75–123.

45. "Claim for an Increased Invalid Pension," Cyrus Davis Pension Record, certificate 51, 242, Pension Application Files Based Upon Service in the Civil War and Spanish American War, Record Group 15, Records of the Veterans Administration, 1783–1985, NARA, Washington, DC. Davis's case is particularly interesting, as the 1880 census indicates that he continued to farm. Whether he was successful, or what happened after this census data was gathered, is unknown. Tenth Census of the United States, 1880. Records of the Bureau of the Census, Record Group 29, Records of the Bureau of the Census, NARA, Washington, DC.

46. Blanck and Millender, "Before Disability Civil Rights," 5.

47. Logue and Blanck, *Race, Ethnicity and Disability*, 73–78.

48. Zechariah Davis Pension Record, Application 741,637, Pension Application Files Based Upon Service in the Civil War and Spanish American War, Record Group 15, Records of the Veterans Administration, 1783–1985, NARA, Washington, DC.

49. For more on racial disparities in the pension system, see Shaffer, *After the Glory*, 119–42.

50. Powell, *Officers of the Army and Navy (Volunteer)*, 70.

51. "Senator Manderson," *Illustrated American*, March 21, 1891. James Tanner eased evidentiary requirements for pensions, and he sometimes encouraged his clerks to approve even questionable cases. Tanner was commissioner of pensions for five months between March and September 1889. See Marten, *America's Corporal*, 110–13.

52. "Senator Manderson," *Illustrated American*, March 21, 1891.

53. "Rich Pension Beggars," *Harrisburg (PA) Patriot*, July 15, 1889.

54. "Senator Manderson," *Illustrated American*, March 21, 1891.

55. "Examining Surgeons Certificate," Murty Brennan Pension File, certificate 250, 569, Pension Application Files Based Upon Service in the Civil War and Spanish American War, Record Group 15, Records of the Veterans Administration, 1783–1985, NARA, Washington, DC.

56. Untitled document, October 11, 1882. Murty Brennan Pension File, certificate 250, 569.

57. Skocpol, *Protecting Soldiers and Mothers*, 121.

58. Allan Nevins, *Grover Cleveland: A Study in Courage* (New York: Dodd, Mead, 1962), 328. In all, Cleveland vetoed over two hundred private pension bills, though this number was still small compared to the huge numbers he did not veto. Cleveland, *Recollections of Grover Cleveland*, 99; Brodsky, *Grover Cleveland*, 183.

59. Brodsky, *Grover Cleveland*, 25–28; Algeo, *President Is a Sick Man*, 23–25; Nevins, *Grover Cleveland*, 51.

60. Nevins, *Grover Cleveland*, 327; "Led a Gallant Charge," in *Deeds of Honor*, 1:99–100.

61. Brodsky, *Grover Cleveland*, 181–89.

62. Deposition C, Abraham Griggs, November 4, 1891, Abraham P. Griggs Pension File, certificate number 688, 275.

63. Deposition C, Abraham Griggs, November 4, 1891, Abraham P. Griggs Pension File, certificate number 688, 275.

64. Deposition C, Abraham Griggs, November 4, 1891, Abraham P. Griggs Pension File, certificate 688, 275.

65. Deposition C, Abraham Griggs, November 4, 1891, Abraham P. Griggs Pension File, certificate 688, 275.

66. R. M. McMorris to Green B. Raum, Commissioner of Pensions, November 6, 1891, Abraham P. Griggs Pension File, certificate 688, 275.

67. Affidavit of Dr. John H. Irwin, Abraham P. Griggs Pension File, certificate 688, 275.

68. This is not to say that no one ever greased the wheels at the Pension Bureau. See Marten, *America's Corporal*, 92–130.

69. *Public Papers of Grover Cleveland*, 96.

70. United States Congress, Report No. 1565, in *Reports of Committees of the Senate of the United States, for the First Session of the Forty-Ninth Congress*. Mrs. Owen may have gotten the pension eventually; the Congressional Receipts and Expenditures from 1888 lists a thirty-six-dollar pension for an Annie Owens. Whether this is the same woman is not clear. United States Congress, *Executive Documents*, 228.

71. United States Congress, Report No. 977, in *Reports of Committees of the Senate of the United States for the First Session of the Fifty-First Congress*. Mrs. Potts and her congressmen took advantage of Cleveland's ouster in 1889 and resubmitted her bill, which was approved. *The Statutes at Large of the United States of America from December 1889 to March 1891* (Washington, Government Printing Office, 1891).

72. *Public Papers of Grover Cleveland*, 407.

73. *Public Papers of Grover Cleveland*, 337–38.

74. "Caldicott, Augustus F.," in *Annual Report of the Adjutant-General of the State of New York*, 24. The soldier was variously listed as Caldicott, Coldecott, and Caldecott in the sources.

75. "Accidental Death—Tamezan Ball," in *Decisions of the Department of the Interior*, ed. Barber, 3:185.

76. *Public Papers of Grover Cleveland*, 333.
77. "An Outrageous Pension Veto," *Indianapolis Journal*, August 13, 1888.
78. Powell, *Chickamauga Campaign*, 640.
79. United States Congress, Report 1026, in *Reports of Committees of the Senate of the United States for the Session of the Forty-Seventh Congress*.
80. "Outrageous Pension Veto," *Indianapolis Journal*, August 13, 1888.
81. *Public Papers of Grover Cleveland*, 375.
82. "Outrageous Pension Veto," *Indianapolis Journal*, August 13, 1888.
83. *Public Papers of Grover Cleveland*, 110.

CHAPTER 6. The Long, Long Years of Misery

1. Lizzie Wilson McWilliams McReynolds to "Dr. White" [W. A. White], December 14, 1905, John D. Wilson case file, Case Records of Patients, 1855–1950, Record Group 418, Records of St. Elizabeths Hospital, NARA, Washington, DC.

2. Lizzie Wilson McWilliams McReynolds to "Dr. Richardson," December 12, 1909, John D. Wilson case file.

3. Arthur Kleinman, Veena Das, and Margaret Locke, eds., introduction to *Social Suffering* (Berkley: University of California Press, 1997), ix. Continuing research on present-day post-traumatic stress disorder shows that it creates a ripple effect radiating out from the suffering soldier to affect family members. Multigenerational trauma can result. See Carlson and Rozek, "PTSD and the Family," National Center for PTSD, United States Department of Veterans Affairs website, http://www.ptsd.va.gov/professional/treatment/family/ptsd-and-the-family.asp. For a historical treatment of generational trauma, see Reagan, "My Daughter was Genetically Drafted with Me," 833–53.

4. On war trauma, see Dean, *Shook Over Hell*; Sommerville, *Aberration of Mind*; Sommerville, "Burden Too Heavy to Bear"; Sommerville, "Will They Ever Be Able to Forget?," in *Weirding the War*, ed. Berry; Belt, "Ballots for Bullets?"; McClurken, *Take Care of the Living*; Silkenat, *Moments of Despair*; Carroll, "God Who Shielded Me Before," 252–80; Marten, *Sing Not War*; Gordon, *A Broken Regiment*. For a response to Civil War trauma scholarship, see Hsieh, "Go to Your Gawd Like a Soldier."

5. Retrospective diagnosis runs the risk of flattening disabled people's complex lived experiences into cut-and-dried medical symptoms and treatments, with very little gained. It also seems to me that focusing on finding the exact diagnosis for Civil War soldiers distracts us from exploring lived experience of disability and disease. For some of the discussions scholars of disability and medical ethics have had on retrospective diagnosis, see Muramoto, "Retrospective Diagnosis," 1–15; Karenberg, "Retrospective Diagnosis," 140–45.

6. While their different roles became blurred late in the century, Utica was intended to be the place for acutely ill patients, while Willard was designed to be a long-term care facility for incurable patients. For the history of the two institutions

160   Notes to Chapter Six

and the context of the nineteenth-century institution, see Dowbiggin, *Keeping America Sane*. During the war, St. Elizabeths was officially named the Government Asylum for the Insane, but it was colloquially known by its nickname. The asylum was officially renamed St. Elizabeths in 1916. See Millikan, "Wards of the Nation," 8. For context on the asylum in nineteenth-century America, see, for example, Tomes, *Art of Asylum-Keeping*; David Rothman, *The Discovery of the Asylum: Social Order and Disorder in the New Republic* (New York: Little, Brown, 1971); Grob, *Mad among Us*; Whitaker, *Mad in America*.

7. It's not clear how many of these letters ever reached their intended recipients. Physicians preserved many of the soldiers' and veterans' letters, and I assume that the communications were intercepted and never sent.

8. Daniel Folsom is a pseudonym, as are the names given for all the soldiers and veterans institutionalized at Utica and the Willard Asylum for the Chronic Insane. In accordance with New York State Mental Hygiene Law 33.13, I have obscured personally identifying information to protect patient privacy. I use real names when discussing soldiers from St. Elizabeths because doing so is not restricted. I refer to the doctors at Utica in vague terms because the doctors adding to patients' case files very rarely included their own names. Daniel Folsom [pseud.] case file, Utica State Hospital Patient Case Files, 1843–1898, New York State Archives, Albany.

9. Thomson, *Historical Sketch of the Sixteenth Regiment*, 12.

10. Daniel Folsom [pseud.] case file.

11. Daniel Folsom [pseud.] case file. It is not always clear which doctor took down patient notes or conducted intakes.

12. Daniel Folsom [pseud.] to Sister, March 2, 1864, Daniel Folsom [pseud.], case file. Spelling in original.

13. Daniel Folsom [pseud.] to Sister, March 2, 1864, Daniel Folsom [pseud.], case file.

14. Gregory Toombs [pseud.] case file, Utica State Hospital Patient Case Files, 1843–1898, New York State Archives, Albany.

15. Gregory Toombs [pseud.] case file.

16. Gregory Toombs [pseud.] to John P. Gray, January 3, 1876, Gregory Toombs [pseud.] case file.

17. Gregory Toombs [pseud.] case file.

18. Benjamin F. Ellis to "Uncle," September 7, 1870, Benjamin F. Ellis case file, Case Records of Patients, 1855–1950, Record Group 418, Records of St. Elizabeths Hospital, NARA, Washington, DC.

19. Benjamin F. Ellis to "Uncle," September 7, 1870. Benjamin F. Ellis case file.

20. Benjamin F. Ellis to "Uncle," September 7, 1870. Benjamin F. Ellis Case File.

21. Charles Danielson [pseud.] patient case file, Utica State Hospital Patient Case Files, 1843–1898, New York State Archives, Albany; *Civil War Muster Roll Abstracts of New York State Volunteers, United States Sharpshooters, and United States*

Colored Troops [ca. 1861–1900], microfilm, 1185 rolls, New York State Archives, Albany.

22. Charles Danielson [pseud.] to "Friends," February 17, 1865, Charles Danielson patient case file.

23. Kinder, *Paying with Their Bodies*, 121. See also Gelber, "Hard Boiled Order," 161–80; Lawrie, "Salvaging the Negro," in *Disability Histories*, ed. Rembis and Burch; Linker, *War's Waste*.

24. Robert Martin [pseud.] case file, Utica State Hospital Patient Case Files, 1843–1898, New York State Archives, Albany.

25. Jeremiah Norris [pseud.] case file, Utica State Hospital Patient Case Files, 1843–1898, New York State Archives, Albany.

26. Jeremiah Norris [pseud.] case file. For more on the links between nineteenth-century psychiatry, masturbation, and sexuality, see Barker-Benfield, "Spermatic Economy,", 45–74; Barker-Benfield, *Horrors of the Half-Known Life*.

27. Edgar Brown [pseud.] case file, Willard State Hospital Patient Case Files, 1869-1938, New York State Archives, Albany.

28. Daniel Folsom [pseud.] to Sister, March 2, 1864, Daniel Folsom [pseud.] case file.

29. *Civil War Muster Roll Abstracts*, microfilm, 1185 rolls.

30. Tenth Census of the United States, 1880.

31. "Robert Martin Retires," *Columbia Republican* (Hudson, NY) January 3, 1908. In accordance with New York State Mental Hygiene Law 33.13, I have changed the title of this newspaper article to reflect the pseudonym I use for this soldier.

32. "Treasury Changes," *Evening Star* (Washington, DC), October 7, 1904.

33. For example, Dean, *Shook Over Hell*; Sommerville, "Burden Too Heavy to Bear"; Sommerville, "Will They Ever Be Able to Forget?"; Silkenat, *Moments of Despair*; McClurken, *Take Care of the Living*.

34. For an excellent analysis of the ways that families of Revolutionary War veterans adapted, see Blackie, "Disability, Dependency, and the Family." For more on the Civil War's impact on families, see for example, Marten, *Children's Civil War*; Bleser and Gordon, *Intimate Strategies of the Civil War*; Taylor, *Divided Family in Civil War America*; Sheehan-Dean, *Why Confederates Fought*; Riley, "This Is the Last Time."

35. Affidavit of Mrs. Maria Kielhoffer, Francis Kielhoffer Pension File, certificate number 625,017, Pension Application Files Based Upon Service in the Civil War and Spanish American War, Record Group 15, Records of the Veterans Administration, 1783–1985, NARA, Washington, DC.

36. Affidavit of Mrs. Maria Kielhoffer, Francis Kielhoffer Pension File, certificate number 625,017.

37. Harriet Kane to "Dear Sir," March 11, 1877. Joseph Zane case file, Case Records of Patients, 1855–1950, Record Group 418, Records of St. Elizabeths Hospital, NARA, Washington, DC.

38. Geoffrey Johnson [pseud.] case file, Utica State Hospital Patient Case Files, New York State Archives, Albany; Isaiah Seaborn [pseud.] case file, Utica State Hospital Case Files, New York State Archives, Albany. Seaborn was eventually transferred to the Willard Asylum for the Chronic Insane, a residential institution for patients not expected to improve. He was never released, and he died in the asylum in 1888 of *phthsis pulmonalis* at age forty-four.

39. Michael Mitchell [pseud.] case file, Willard State Hospital Patient Case Files, 1869-1938, New York State Archives, Albany; Abstracts from Original Muster Rolls for New York State Infantry Units Involved in the Civil War, New York State Archives, Albany.

40. Jacob Kyle [pseud.] patient case files, Willard State Hospital Patient Case Files, 1869–1938, New York State Archives, Albany.

41. Affidavit of Mrs. Maria Kielhoffer, Francis Kielhoffer Pension File, certificate number 625, 017.

42. William Brenton [pseud.] case file, Utica State Hospital Patient Case Files, 1843–1898, New York State Archives, Albany.

43. Clinton Moore [pseud.] case file, Utica State Hospital Patient Case Files, 1843–1898, New York State Archives, Albany.

44. Clinton Moore [pseud.] case file.

45. Robert Martin [pseud.] case file.

46. Mrs. M. M. Ellis to Charles Nichols, May 19, 1872, Benjamin F. Ellis case file.

47. James Wright to "The Superintendent of the Insane Institution," January 6, 1886, Jonathan Wright case file, Case Records of Patients, 1855–1950, Record Group 418, Records of St. Elizabeths Hospital, NARA, Washington, DC.

48. Samuel Whiteside case file, Case Records of Patients, 1855–1950, Record Group 418, Records of St. Elizabeths Hospital, NARA, Washington, DC.

49. C. W. Moncrief to W. W. Godding, November 25, 1886, John T. Moncrief case file, Case Records of Patients, 1855–1950, Record Group 418, Records of St. Elizabeths Hospital, NARA, Washington, DC; Tenth Census of the United States, 1880.

50. Dennis Hammifin to "My Doctor Nickle" [Dr. Nichols], July 29, 1891, Timothy Hammifin case file, Case Records of Patients, 1855–1950, Record Group 418, Records of St. Elizabeths Hospital, NARA, Washington, DC.

51. Dennis Hammifin to "Dear Sir," November 28, 1893, Timothy Hammifin case file.

52. Mrs. Mary Carty to "Honored Sir," February 1, 1886, David Carty case file, Case Records of Patients, 1855–1950, Record Group 418, Records of St. Elizabeths Hospital, NARA, Washington, DC.

53. Maria Sine to "Mr. Nichols," undated, Henry Gibson case file, Case Records of Patients, 1855–1950, Record Group 418, Records of St. Elizabeths Hospital, NARA, Washington, DC.

54. Maria Sine to "Mr. Nichols," undated, Henry Gibson case file.

55. Mrs. Lizzie H. Stoner to W. A. White, October 21, 1904, Franklin B. Hayes case file, Case Records of Patients, 1855–1950, Record Group 418, Records of St. Elizabeths Hospital, NARA, Washington, DC.

56. Mrs. Lizzie H. Stoner to unknown, undated, Franklin B. Hayes case file.

57. E. Alford Bush to "The Supt of the Govt Hospital," January 27, 1888, Norton C. Bush case files, Case Records of Patients, 1855–1950, Record Group 418, Records of St. Elizabeths Hospital, NARA, Washington, DC.

58. Mrs. J. C. Rue to "Supt. of Insane Asylum" [W. W. Godding], June 10, 1879, John Ira Rue case file, Case Records of Patients, 1855–1950, Record Group 418, Records of St. Elizabeths Hospital, NARA, Washington, DC.

59. Lizzie Wilson McWilliams McReynolds to W. W. Godding, September 18 (no year), John D. Wilson case file.

60. Lizzie Wilson McWilliams McReynolds to W. W. Godding, February 24, 1887, John D. Wilson case file.

61. Lizzie Wilson McReynolds to W. W. Godding, December 21, 1878, John D. Wilson case file.

62. Lizzie Wilson McWilliams McReynolds to A. B. Richardson, December 13, 1900, John D. Wilson case file.

63. Lizzie Wilson McWilliams McReynolds to "Supt Gov. Hsptl," June 20, 1900, John D. Wilson case file.

64. Lizzie Wilson McWilliams McReynolds to "Supt Gov. Hsptl," June 20, 1900, John D. Wilson case file.

65. David C. Wilson to W. W. Godding, April 14, 1893, John D. Wilson case file.

66. Lizzie Wilson McWilliams McReynolds to Mr. Richardson, December 18, 1909, John D. Wilson case file.

67. Lizzie Wilson McWilliams McReynolds to W. W. White, December 1911, John D. Wilson case file.

68. Daniel Folsom [pseud.] case file. Spelling in original.

EPILOGUE

1. Rachel Feltman, "Wounded Soldier Set to Receive the First Penis Transplant in U.S.," *Washington Post*, February 18, 2016; Quil Lawrence, "For Fertility Treatment, Wounded Veterans Have to Pay the Bill," National Public Radio (hereafter NPR), February 17, 2016, https://www.npr.org/sections/health-shots/2016/02/17/467073198/for-fertility-treatment-wounded-veterans-have-to-foot-the-bill.

2. See the series of investigations done by Quil Lawrence and Marisa Peñaloza: "Filling the Gaps for Veterans with Bad Discharges," NPR, December 12, 2013, https://www.npr.org/2013/12/12/250289588/filling-the-gaps-for-veterans-with-bad-discharges; "Path to Reclaiming Identity Steep for Vets with 'Bad Paper,'" NPR, December 11, 2013, https://www.npr.org/2013/12/11/249962933/path-to-reclaiming

-identity-steep-for-vets-with-bad-paper; "Other-Than-Honorable Discharge Burdens Like a Scarlet Letter," NPR, December 9, 2013, https://www.npr.org/2013/12/09/249342610/other-than-honorable-discharge-burdens-like-a-scarlet-letter.

3. Sarah Handley-Cousins, "How Work Requirements for Medicaid Hurt People with 'Invisible' Disabilities," Made by History, *Washington Post*, January 18, 2018.

4. "Insult to Injury: America's Vanishing Worker Protections," NPR and *ProPublica*, 2015, https://www.npr.org/series/394891172/insult-to-injury-americas-vanishing-worker-protections.

BIBLIOGRAPHY

Manuscript Collections

Alice Rains Trulock Papers, Pejepscot Historical Society, Brunswick, ME.
Case Files of Approved Pension Applications of Widows and Other Dependents of the Army and Navy Who Served Mainly in the Civil War and the War With Spain, Record Group 15, Records of the Veterans Administration, 1861–1934, National Archives and Records Administration, Washington, DC.
Case Records of Patients, 1855–1950, Record Group 418, Records of St. Elizabeths Hospital, National Archives and Records Administration, Washington, DC.
Chamberlain-Adams Collection, Radcliffe College Schlesinger Library.
Court-Martial Case Files and Related Records, Record Group 153, Records of the Office of the Judge Advocate General (Army), 1792–2010, National Archives and Records Administration, Washington, DC.
Henry A. Barnum Collection, Onondaga Historical Association, Syracuse, NY.
Joshua Lawrence Chamberlain Collection, Bowdoin College Special Collections, Brunswick, ME.
Joshua Lawrence Chamberlain Collection, Pejepscot Historical Society, Brunswick, ME.
Joshua Lawrence Chamberlain Medical File, Pejepscot Historical Society, Brunswick, ME.
Levy Sheet Music Collection, Johns Hopkins Sheridan Libraries and University Museums.
Pension Application Files Based Upon Service in the Civil War and Spanish American War, Record Group 15, Records of the Veterans Administration, 1783–1985, National Archives and Records Administration, Washington, DC.
Proceedings of the Board Established to Examine Officers of the Veteran Reserve Corps and Applicants for Appointment to the Corps, 1864–1865, Records of the Provost Marshal General's Bureau, Record Group 110, National Archives and Records Administration, Washington, DC.
Surgical Photographs, 1860s–1880s, Otis Historical Archives, National Museum of Health and Medicine, Silver Spring, MD.
Tenth Census of the United States, Record Group 29, Records of the Bureau of the Census, National Archives and Records Administration, Washington, DC.

Utica State Hospital Patient Case Files, 1843–1898, New York State Archives.
Willard State Hospital Patient Case Files, 1869–1938, New York State Archives.
William Henry Noble Papers, Duke University Rubenstein Library, Durham, NC.

Periodicals

Albany (NY) Journal
Appleton's Journal
Army and Navy Journal and Gazette of the Regular and Volunteer Forces, Vol. II 1864–1865
Bedford (PA) Gazette
Boston Journal
Cincinnati Gazette
Cleveland Leader
Daily Herald (Grand Forks, ND)
Daily Inter Ocean (Chicago, IL)
Daily Register (Sandusky, OH)
Farmer's Cabinet (Amherst, NH)
Godey's Magazine
Harper's Weekly
Harrisburg (PA) Patriot
Hearst's Magazine
Illustrated American
Indianapolis Journal
Jackson (MI) Citizen
Jersey Journal (Hudson County, NJ)
Kansas City (KA) Times
Lippincott's Magazine of Literature, Science and Education
National American (Bel Air, MD)
New York Herald
New York Observer & Chronicle
New York Sun
New York Times
New York Tribune
Portland (ME) Transcript
Portland Oregonian
St. Louis Republic
Syracuse Courier
Times-Picayune (New Orleans, LA)
Washington Star (Washington, DC)
Weekly Telegraph (Macon, GA)
World (New York, NY)

Printed Primary Sources

Ames, Mary Clemmer. *Ten Years in Washington: Life and Scenes in the National Capital, as a Woman Sees Them.* Cincinnati: Queen City Publishing, 1874.

Annual Report of the Adjutant-General of the State of New York for the Year 1900. Albany: J.B. Lyon, 1902.

Bailey, Judith A., and Robert I. Cottom, eds. *After Chancellorsville: Letters from the Heart.* Baltimore: Maryland Historical Society, 1998.

Barber, George, ed. *Decisions of the Department of the Interior in Cases Relating to Pension Claims and to the Laws of the United States Granting and Governing Pensions, with Appendix.* Volume 3. Washington, DC: Government Printing Office, 1890.

Barnes, Joseph K. et al., eds. *The Medical and Surgical History of the War of the Rebellion.* Part 1, Vol. 1. Washington, DC: Government Printing Office, 1870.

———. *The Medical and Surgical History of the War of the Rebellion,* Part 2, Vol. 2. Washington, DC: Government Printing Office, 1888.

Bartholow, Roberts. *A Manual of Instructions for Enlisting and Discharging Soldiers, With Special Reference to the Medical Examination of Recruits and the Detection of Disqualification and Feigned Diseases.* Philadelphia: J. B. Lippincott, 1863.

Beyer, Walter and Oscar Keydel. *Deeds of Honor: From Records in the Archives of the United States Government, How American Heroes Won the Medal of Honor.* Vol. 1. Detroit: Perrien-Keydel, 1907.

Billings, John Shaw. *Medical Museums, with Special Reference to the Army Medical Museum at Washington.* Medical News, 1888.

Brinton, John H. *Personal Memoirs of John H. Brinton, Major and Surgeon, U.S.V., 1861–1865.* New York: Neale, 1914.

Chamberlain, Joshua Lawrence. *The Passing of the Armies: An Account of the Final Campaign of the Army of the Republic.* 1915. Lincoln: University of Nebraska Press, 1998.

Child, William. *A History of the Fifth Regiment, New Hampshire Volunteers, in the American Civil War, 1861–1865.* Bristol: R. W. Musgrave, 1893.

Cleveland, Grover. *Recollections of Grover Cleveland.* Edited by George Frederick Parker. New York: Century, 1909.

———. *The Public Papers of Grover Cleveland, Twenty-Second President of the United States, March 4, 1885, to March 4, 1889.* Washington, DC: Government Printing Office, 1889.

Donald, David Herbert, ed., *Gone for a Soldier: The Civil War Memories of Private Alfred Bellard.* Boston: Little Brown, 1975.

Eliot, Charles. *President Eliot's Speech at the Bay State Club, Oct. 12, 1889.* Boston: Young Men's Democratic Club of Mass., 1889.

Field Record of the Officers of the Veteran Reserve Corps, from the Commencement to the Close of the Rebellion. Washington: Scrivner and Swing, 1865.

Grace, William. *The Army Surgeon's Manual, for the Use of Medical Officers, Cadets, Chaplains and Hospital Stewards*. New York: Bailliere Brothers, 1864.

Holmes, Oliver Wendell. *Soundings from the Atlantic*. Boston: Ticknor and Fields, 1864.

McCarthy, Carlton. *Detailed Minutiae of Soldier Life in the Army of Northern Virginia, 1861–1865*. Richmond: Carlton McCarthy, 1882.

Moore, Frank, ed. *The Rebellion Record: A Diary of American Events*. New York: G. P. Putnam, 1863.

Moore, John. *The Medical and Surgical History of the War of the Rebellion*. Part 3, Vol. 1. Washington, DC: Government Printing Office, 1888.

Philadelphia College of Pharmacy Alumni Report. Vol. 28, p. 200. Philadelphia: Alumni Association of the Philadelphia College of Pharmacy, 1891.

Powell, William H. *Officers of the Army and Navy (Volunteer) Who Served in the Civil War*. Philadelphia: L. R. Hamersley, 1893.

Roosevelt, Theodore. *The Strenuous Life: Essays and Addresses*. New York: Century, 1902.

Scribner, B. F. *How Soldiers Were Made: Or, the War as I Saw It Under Buell, Rosecrans, Thomas, Grant, and Sherman*. Chicago: Donohue and Henneberry, 1887.

Stowe, Harriet Beecher. *Uncle Tom's Cabin*. London: John Cassel, Ludgate Hall, 1852.

Sturgis, Thomas. *Prisoners of War, 1861–1865*. New York: G.P. Putnam's Sons, 1912.

Thomson, William H. *Historical Sketch of the Sixteenth Regiment, N.Y.S. Volunteer Infantry, April 1861–May 1863*. Albany, 1880.

United States Congress. *The Executive Documents of the House of Representatives for the Second Session of the Fifty-First Congress, 1890–1891*. Washington, DC: Government Printing Office, 1891.

———. *Reports of Committees of the Senate of the United States for the First Session of the Fifty-First Congress, 1889–1890*. Washington, DC: Government Printing Office, 1891.

———. *Reports of Committees of the Senate of the United States, for the First Session of the Forty-Ninth Congress, 1885–1886*. Washington, DC: Government Printing Office, 1886.

———. *Reports of Committees of the Senate of the United States for the Session of the Forty-Seventh Congress, 1882–1883*. Washington, DC: Government Printing Office, 1883.

United States Sanitary Commission. *Hospital Transports: A Memoir of the Embarkation of the Sick and Wounded from the Peninsula of Virginia in the Summer of 1862*. Boston: Ticknor and Fields, 1863.

United States War Department. *United States Army Regulations of 1861*. Washington, DC: Government Printing Office, 1865.

———. *The War of the Rebellion: A Compilation of the Official Records of the Union and Confederate Armies*. 128 vols. Washington, DC: Government Printing Office, 1880–1901.

Secondary Literature

Adam, Daniel. *The Unwritten War: American Writers and the Civil War*. New York: Knopf, 1973.
Adams, Buford. *E Pluribus Barnum: The Great Showman and the Making of U.S. Popular Culture*. Minneapolis: University of Minnesota Press, 1997.
Adams, John Worthington. *Doctors in Blue: The Medical History of the Union Army in the Civil War*. New York: H. Schuman, 1952.
Albrecht, Gary, Katherine Seelman, and Michael Bury, eds. *Handbook of Disability Studies*. Thousand Oaks, CA: Sage, 2001.
Algeo, Matthew. *The President Is a Sick Man: Wherein the Supposedly Virtuous Grover Cleveland Survives a Secret Surgery at Sea and Vilifies the Courageous Newspaperman Who Dared Expose the Truth*. Chicago: Chicago Review Press, 2011.
Anderson, Donald Lee, and Godfrey Tryggve Anderson. "Nostalgia and Malingering in the Military during the Civil War." *Perspectives in Biology and Medicine* 28, no. 1 (1984): 156–66.
Barbian, Lenore, Paul S. Sledzik, and Jeffrey S. Resznick. "Remains of War: Walt Whitman, Civil War Soldiers, and the Legacy of Medical Collections." *Museum History Journal* 5, no. 1 (2012): 7–28.
Barker-Benfield, G. John. *The Horrors of the Half-Known Life: Male Attitudes toward Women and Sexuality in Nineteenth-Century America*. New York: Routledge, 2000.
———. "The Spermatic Economy: A Nineteenth Century View of Sexuality." *Feminist Studies* 1 (Summer 1972): 45–74.
Barnes, Colin, and Geoff Mercer, eds. *Exploring the Divide: Illness and Disability*. Leeds: Disability Press, 1996.
Baynton, Douglas. "Disability as a Justification for Inequality in American History," in *The New Disability History*, edited by Paul K. Longmore and Laurel Umansky, 33–57. New York: New York University Press, 2001.
Bederman, Gail. *Manliness & Civilization: A Cultural History of Gender and Race in the United States, 1880–1917*. Chicago: University of Chicago Press, 1995.
Beilein, Joseph M., Jr. "The Guerrilla Shirt: A Labor of Love and the Style of Rebellion in Civil War Missouri." *Civil War History* 58 (June 2012): 151–79.
Belt, Rabia. "Ballots for Bullets? Disabled Veterans and the Right to Vote." *Stanford Law Review* 69 (February 2017): 435–90.
Blackie, Daniel. "Disability, Dependency, and the Family in the Early United States in Disability Histories," in *Disability Histories*, edited by Michael Rembis and Susan Burch, 17–35. Urbana: University of Illinois Press, 2014.
Blair, William. *Cities of the Dead: Contesting the Memory of the Civil War in the South, 1865–1914*. Chapel Hill: University of North Carolina Press, 2004.
Blakeley, Robert L., and Judith M. Harrington. *Bones in the Basement: Post-Mortem Racism in Nineteenth-Century Medical Training*. Washington, DC: Smithsonian Institution Press, 1997.

Blanck, Peter David, and Michael Millender. "Before Disability Civil Rights: Pensions and the Politics of Disability in America." *Alabama Law Review* 52 (2000): 1–50.

Bleser, Carol K., and Lesley J. Gordon, eds. *Intimate Strategies of the Civil War: Military Commanders and Their Wives.* Oxford: Oxford University Press, 2001.

Blight, David. *Race and Reunion: The Civil War in American Memory.* Cambridge, MA: Harvard University Press, 2001.

Bollett, Alfred. *Civil War Medicine: Challenges and Triumphs.* Tucson: Galen, 2002.

Boster, Dea H. "'Unfit for Ordinary Purposes': Disability, Slaves, and Decision Making in the Antebellum American South," in *Disability Histories*, edited by Michael Rembis and Susan Burch, 201–18. Urbana: University of Illinois Press, 2014.

Bourrier, Karen. *The Measure of Manliness: Disability and Masculinity in the Mid-Victorian Novel.* Ann Arbor: University of Michigan Press, 2015.

Brodsky, Alyn. *Grover Cleveland: A Study in Character.* New York: Truman Talley Books, St. Martin's, 2000.

Carroll, Dillon J. "'The God Who Shielded Me Before, Yet Watches Over Us All': Confederate Soldiers, Mental Illness, and Religion." *Civil War History* 61 (2015): 252–80.

Casey, John A., Jr. "Marked by War: Demobilization, Disability, and the Trope of the Citizen-Soldier in *Miss Ravenel's Conversion.*" *Civil War History* 60 (2014): 123–51.

———. *New Men: Reconstructing the Image of the Veteran in Late Nineteenth-Century American Literature and Culture.* New York: Fordham University Press, 2015.

Cashin, Joan. "Deserters, Civilians, and Draft Resistance in the North," in *The War Was You and Me: Civilians in the American Civil War*, edited by Joan Cashin, 262–86. Princeton, NJ: Princeton University Press, 2002.

Castel, Albert, ed. "Many . . . Diseases Are . . . Feigned." *Civil War Times Illustrated* 16 (August 1977): 29–32.

Cimbala, Paul A. "Federal Manpower Needs and the U.S. Army's Veteran Reserve Corps," in *Scraping the Barrel: The Military Use of Substandard Manpower, 1860–1960*, edited by Sanders Marble, 5–28. New York: Fordham University Press, 2012.

———. *Veterans North and South: The Transition from Soldier to Civilian After the Civil War.* Santa Barbara: Praeger, 2015.

Clarke, Frances. "So Lonesome I Could Die: Nostalgia and Debates Over Emotional Control in the Civil War North." *Journal of Social History* 41 (2007):253–82.

———. *War Stories: Suffering and Sacrifice in the Civil War North.* Chicago: University of Chicago Press, 2011.

Connor, J. T. H., and Michael G. Rhode. "Shooting Soldiers: Civil War Medical Images, Memory, and Identity in America." *InVisible Culture* 5 (2003).

Cooper Owens, Deirdre. *Medical Bondage: Race, Gender, and the Origins of American Gynecology*. Athens: University of Georgia Press, 2017.
Costa, Dora L. "Changing Chronic Disease Rates and Long-Term Functional Limitation among Older Men," *Demography* 39 (February 2002): 119–37.
———. "Understanding Mid-Life and Older Age Mortality Declines: Evidence from Union Army Veterans." Working Paper 8000, National Bureau of Economic Research, Cambridge, MA, 2000.
Costa, Dora L., and Matthew E. Kahn. *Heroes & Cowards: The Social Face of War*. Princeton, NJ: Princeton University Press, 2008.
———. *The Evolution of Retirement: An American Economic History, 1880–1990*. Chicago: University of Chicago Press, 1998.
Crane, Susan A. "Curious Cabinets and Imaginary Museums," in *Museums and Memory*, edited by Susan A. Crane, 60–81. Stanford, CA: Stanford University Press, 2000.
Cresswell, Tim. *The Tramp in America*. London: Reaktion Books, 2001.
Cullen, Jim. "'I's a Man Now': Gender and African American Men," in *Divided Houses: Gender and the Civil War*, edited by Catherine Clinton and Nina Silber, 76–91. Oxford: Oxford University Press, 1992.
Cunningham, H. H. *Doctors in Gray: The Confederate Medical Service*. Baton Rouge: Louisiana State University Press, 1958.
Daen, Laurel. "Revolutionary War Invalid Pensions and the Bureaucratic Language of Disability in the Early Republic." *Early American Literature* 52 (2017): 141–67.
Davis, N. Ann. "Invisible Disability." *Ethics* 116 (2005): 153–213.
Dean, Eric T. *Shook Over Hell: Post-Traumatic Stress Disorder, Vietnam, and the Civil War*. Cambridge, MA: Harvard University Press, 1997.
DePastino, Todd. *Citizen Hobo: How a Century of Homelessness Shaped America*. Chicago: University of Chicago Press, 2003.
Devine, Shauna. *Learning from the Wounded: The Civil War and the Rise of American Medical Science*. Chapel Hill: University of North Carolina Press, 2014.
Doctorow, E. L. *The March*. New York: Random House, 2005.
Dowbiggin, Ian. *Keeping America Sane: Psychiatry and Eugenics in the United States and Canada, 1880–1940*. Ithaca, NY: Cornell University Press, 1997.
Downs, Jim. *Sick from Freedom: African American Illness and Suffering during the Civil War and Reconstruction*. Oxford: Oxford University Press, 2012.
Du Bois, W. E. B. *The Souls of Black Folk*. Chicago: McClurg, 1903.
Dunkelman, Mark. *Brothers One and All: Espirit de Corps in a Civil War Regiment*. Baton Rouge: Louisiana State University Press, 2004.
Edwards, Rebecca. *New Spirits: Americans in the Gilded Age, 1865–1905*. Oxford: Oxford University Press, 2006.
Ehrenreich, Barbara, and Dierdre English. *For Her Own Good: Two Centuries of Experts' Advice to Women*. New York: Anchor Books, 1978.

Emberton, Carole. "'Only Murder Makes Men': Reconsidering the Black Military Experience." *Journal of the Civil War Era* 2 (2012): 369–93.

Essah, Patience. *A House Divided: Slavery and Emancipation in Delaware, 1638–1865*. Charlottesville: University of Virginia Press, 1996.

Fabian, Ann. *The Skull Collectors: Race, Science, and America's Unburied Dead*. Chicago: University of Chicago Press, 2010.

Faden, Ruth R., and Tom L. Beauchamp. *History and Theory of Informed Consent*. Oxford: Oxford University Press, 1986.

Fahs, Alice. *The Imagined Civil War: Popular Literature of the North and South, 1861–1865*. Chapel Hill: University of North Carolina Press, 2001.

Faust, Drew Gilpin. *Mothers of Invention: Women of the Slaveholding South*. Chapel Hill: University of North Carolina Press, 1996.

———. *This Republic of Suffering: Death and the American Civil War*. New York: Knopf, 2008.

Fellman, Michael. *Inside War: The Guerrilla Conflict in Missouri during the American Civil War*. Oxford: Oxford University Press, 1990.

Fett, Sharla. *Working Cures: Healing, Health and Power on Southern Slave Plantations*. Chapel Hill: University of North Carolina Press, 2002.

Foote, Lorien. *The Gentlemen and the Roughs: Violence, Honor, and Manhood in the Union Army*. New York: New York University Press, 2010.

Fraser, Nancy, and Linda Gordon. "A Genealogy of Dependency: Tracing a Keyword of the U.S. Welfare State." *Signs* 19 (1994): 309–36.

Frawley, Maria H. *Invalidism and Identity in Nineteenth-Century Britain*. Chicago: University of Chicago Press, 2004.

Freemon, Frank. *Gangrene and Glory: Medical Care during the American Civil War*. Madison, NJ: Fairleigh Dickinson University Press, 1998.

Fry, Gladys-Marie. *Night Riders in Black Folk History*. Knoxville: University of Tennessee Press, 1975.

Gallagher, Gary W. *The Union War*. Cambridge, MA: Harvard University Press, 2011.

Gallagher, Gary W., and Kathryn Shively Meier. "Coming to Terms with Military History." *Journal of the Civil War Era* 4 (2014): 487–508.

Gannon, Barbara. *The Won Cause: Black and White Comradeship in the Grand Army of the Republic*. Chapel Hill: University of North Carolina Press, 2011.

Gelber, Scott. "'The Hard Boiled Order': The Reeducation of Disabled WWI Veterans in New York City." *Journal of Social History* 39 (2005): 161–80.

Glatthaar, Joseph T. *Forged in Battle: The Civil War Alliance of Black Soldiers and White Officers*. New York: Free Press, 1990.

Goldberg, Chad. *Citizens and Paupers: Relief, Rights, and Race from the Freedmen's Bureau to Workfare*. Chicago: University of Chicago Press, 2007.

Goler, Robert I., and Michael G. Rhode. "From Individual Trauma to National Policy: Tracking the Uses of Civil War Veteran Medical Records," in *Disabled Veterans in History*, edited by David Gerber, 163–85. Ann Arbor: University of Michigan Press, 2000.

Gordon, Lesley. *A Broken Regiment: The 16th Connecticut's Civil War*. Baton Rouge: Louisiana State University Press, 2014.

Gorn, Elliott. *The Manly Art: Bare-Knuckle Prize Fighting in America*. Ithaca, NY: Cornell University Press, 1986.

Gould, Stephen Jay. *The Mismeasure of Man*. Revised and expanded ed. New York: W. W. Norton, 1996.

Grant, Susan-Mary. "Citizen-Soldiers, Disabled Veterans, and Confederate Nationalism in the Age of People's War." *Journal of the Civil War Era* 2 (2012): 233–54.

Greenberg, Amy S. *Manifest Manhood and the Antebellum American Empire*. Cambridge: Cambridge University Press, 2005.

Greenberg, Kenneth. *Honor and Slavery: Lies, Duels, Noses, Masks, Dressing as a Woman, Gifts, Strangers, Humanitarianism, Death, Slave Rebellions, the Proslavery Argument, Baseball, Hunting, and Gambling in the Old South*. Princeton, NJ: Princeton University Press, 1996.

Grob, Gerald. *The Mad among Us: A History of the Case of America's Mentally Ill*. New York: Free Press, 1994.

Hacker, J. David. "A Census-Based Count of the Civil War Dead." *Civil War History* 57 (December 2011): 307–48.

Hardesty, Ross. *Unfreedom: Slavery and Dependence in Eighteenth-Century Boston*. New York: New York University Press, 2016.

Harmon, William J., and Charles K. McAllister. "The Lion of the Union: The Pelvic Wound of Joshua Lawrence Chamberlain." *Journal of Urology* 163 (2000): 713–16.

Harrison, Simon. *Dark Trophies: Hunting the Enemy Body in Modern War*. New York: Berghahn Books, 2012.

Harsh, Joseph L. *Taken at the Flood: Robert E. Lee and the Maryland Campaign of 1862*. Kent, OH: Kent State University Press, 1999.

Hasegawa, Guy R. *Mending Broken Soldiers: The Union and Confederate Programs to Supply Artificial Limbs*. Carbondale: Southern Illinois University Press, 2012.

Herr, Harry. "'The Privates Were Shot': Urological Wounds and Treatment in the Civil War," in *Years of Change and Suffering: Modern Perspectives on Civil War Medicine*, edited by James M. Schmidt and Guy R. Hasegawa, 89–106. Roseville, MN: Edinburgh Press, 2009.

Herschbach, Lisa. "Fragmentation and Reunion: Medicine, Memory, and Body in the American Civil War." PhD diss., Harvard University, 1997.

Hess, Earl J. *Liberty, Virtue, and Progress: Northerners and Their War for the Union*. New York: Fordham University Press, 1997.

———. *The Union Soldier in Battle: Enduring the Ordeal of Battle*. Lawrence: University of Kansas Press, 1997.

———. "Where Do We Stand? A Critical Assessment of Civil War Studies in the Sesquicentennial." *Civil War History* 60 (2014): 371–403.

Hill, Daniel Delis. *American Menswear: From the Civil War to the Twenty-First Century*. Lubbock: Texas Tech University Press, 2011.

Hoganson, Kristin L. *Fighting for American Manhood: How Gender Politics Provoked the Spanish-American and Philippine-American Wars*. New Haven, CT: Yale University Press, 2000.

Horowitz, Allan. *Creating Mental Illness*. Chicago: University of Chicago Press, 2003.

Howe, Daniel Walker. *What Hath God Wrought: The Transformation of America, 1815–1848*. Oxford: Oxford University Press, 2007.

Hsieh, Wayne Wei-Siang. "'Go to Your Gawd Like a Soldier': Transnational Reflections on Veteranhood." *Journal of the Civil War Era* 5 (December 2015): 551–77.

Humphreys, Margaret. *Intensely Human: The Health of the Black Soldier in the American Civil War*. Baltimore: Johns Hopkins University Press, 2008.

———. *The Marrow of Tragedy: The Health Crisis of the American Civil War*. Baltimore: Johns Hopkins University Press, 2013.

Janney, Caroline. *Burying the Dead but Not the Past: Ladies' Memorial Associations & The Lost Cause*. Chapel Hill: University of North Carolina Press, 2008.

———. *Remembering the Civil War: Reunion and the Limits of Reconciliation*. Chapel Hill: University of North Carolina Press, 2013.

Jefferson, Robert F. "'Enabled Courage': Race, Disability, and Black World War II Veterans in Postwar America." *Historian* 65 (2003): 1102–24.

Johnson, Charles F. *The Civil War Letters of Colonel Charles F. Johnson*. Edited by Fred Pelka. Amherst: University of Massachusetts Press, 2004.

Johnson, Paul E. *Sam Patch, the Famous Jumper*. New York: Hill and Wang, 2003.

Johnstone, David. *An Introduction to Disability Studies*. London: Routledge, 2012.

Jones, Jonathan. "The Great Risk of Opium Eating: Physicians Confront Opiate Addiction in the Civil War Era." Paper presented at the Society of Civil War Historians Meeting, Pittsburgh, PA, June 2, 2018.

Jordan, Brian Matthew. "Living Monuments: Union Veteran Amputees and Embodied Memory of the Civil War." *Civil War History* (June 2011): 121–52.

———. *Marching Home: Union Veterans and Their Unending Civil War*. New York: Liveright, 2015.

Jordan, Winthrop. *White Over Black: American Attitudes toward the Negro, 1550–1812*. Chapel Hill: University of North Carolina Press, 1968.

Karenberg, Axel. "Retrospective Diagnosis: Use and Abuse in Medical Historiography." *Prague Medical Report* 110 (2009): 140–45.

Kasson, John F. *Houdini, Tarzan, and the Perfect Man: The White Male Body and the Challenge of Modernity in America*. New York: Hill and Wang, 2001.

Katz, Michael B. *In the Shadow of the Poorhouse: A Social History of Welfare in America*. Revised and expanded ed. New York: Basic Books, 1996.

Kinder, John. *Paying with Their Bodies: American War and the Problem of the Disabled Veteran*. Chicago: University of Chicago Press, 2015.

Kohl, Rhonda M. "'This Godforsaken Town': Death and Disease at Helena, Arkansas, 1862–1863." *Civil War History* 50 (2004): 109–44.

Lande, R. Gregory. *Madness, Malingering, and Malfeasance: The Transformation of Psychiatry and the Law in the Civil War Era*. Washington, DC: Potomac Books, 2005.

Lawrie, Paul. "'Salvaging the Negro': Race, Rehabilitation, and the Body Politic in World War I America, 1917–1924," in *Disability Histories*, edited by Mike Rembis and Susan Burch, 321–45. Urbana: University of Illinois Press, 2014.

Lenker, Christian. *The Civil War Memoir of Sgt. Christian Lenker, 19th Ohio Volunteers*. Edited by Michael Barton and Judith A. Kennedy. Bloomington: Xlibris, 2014.

Linderman, Gerald. *Embattled Courage: The Experience of Combat in the American Civil War*. New York: Free Press, 1987.

Linker, Beth. *War's Waste: Rehabilitation in World War I America*. Chicago: University of Chicago Press, 2011.

Logue, Larry M., and Peter Blanck. *Race, Ethnicity and Disability: Veterans and Benefits in Post–Civil War America*. Cambridge: Cambridge University Press, 2010.

Longmore, Paul K., and Lauri Urmansky, eds. *The New Disability History: American Perspectives*. New York: New York University Press, 2001.

Lonn, Ella. *Desertion during the Civil War*. New York: Century, 1928.

Lott, Eric. *Love and Theft: Blackface Minstrelsy and the American Working Class*. Oxford: Oxford University Press, 1993.

Lowry, Thomas P., and Jack D. Welsh. *Tarnished Scalpels: The Court-Martials of Fifty Union Surgeons*. Mechanicsburg, PA: Stackpole Books, 2000.

Marshall, Nicholas. "The Great Exaggeration: Death and the Civil War." *Journal of the Civil War Era* 4 (2014): 3–27.

Marten, James. *America's Corporal: James Tanner in War and Peace*. Athens: University of Georgia Press, 2014.

———. *The Children's Civil War*. Chapel Hill: University of North Carolina Press, 1998.

———. "Nomads in Blue: Disabled Veterans and Alcohol at the National Home," in *Disabled Veterans in History*, edited by Daniel Gerber, 275–95. Ann Arbor: University of Michigan Press, 2012.

———. *Sing Not War: The Lives of Union & Confederate Veterans in Gilded Age America*. Chapel Hill: University of North Carolina Press, 2011.

McAllister, Charles K. "Fire, Blood, and the Lion of the Union: Joshua Lawrence Chamberlain's Civil War Ailments." *Pharos of Alpha Omega Alpha Honor Medical Society* 61 (1998): 713–16.

McClurken, Jeffrey W. *Take Care of the Living: Reconstructing Confederate Veteran Families in Virginia*. Charlottesville: University of Virginia Press, 2009.

McConnell, Stuart. *Glorious Contentment: The Grand Army of the Republic, 1865–1890*. Chapel Hill: University of North Carolina Press, 1992.

McCurry, Stephanie. *Masters of Small Worlds: Yeoman Households, Gender Relations, and the Political Culture of the Antebellum South Carolina Low Country*. Cambridge: Oxford University Press, 1997.

McPherson, James. *For Cause and Comrades: Why Men Fought in the Civil War*. New York: Oxford University Press, 1997.

———. *What They Fought For, 1861–1865*. Baton Rouge: Louisiana State University Press, 1994.

Meier, Kathryn Shively. *Nature's Civil War: Common Soldiers and the Environment in 1862 Virginia*. Chapel Hill: University of North Carolina Press, 2013.

Mezurek, Kelly. "'De Bottom Rails on Top Now': Black Union Guards and Confederate Prisoners of War," in *Civil War Prisons II*, edited by Michael P. Gray. Kent, OH: Kent State University Press, forthcoming.

Miller, Brian Craig. *Empty Sleeves: Amputation in the Civil War South*. Athens: University of Georgia Press, 2015.

Millikan, Frank R. "Wards of the Nation: The Making of St. Elizabeths Hospital, 1852–1920." PhD diss., George Washington University, 1989.

Mitchell, Laura Remson. "Beyond the Supercrip Syndrome." *Quill* 77 (1989): 18–23.

Mitchell, Reid. *The Vacant Chair: The Northern Soldier Leaves Home*. Oxford: Oxford University Press, 1993.

Muramoto, Osamu. "Retrospective Diagnosis of a Famous Historical Figure: Ontological, Epistemic, and Ethical Considerations." *Philosophy, Ethics, and Humanities in Medicine* 9 (2014): 10–25.

Neff, John R. *Honoring the Civil War Dead: Commemoration and the Problem of Reconciliation*. Lawrence: University of Kansas Press, 2005.

Nelson, Megan Kate. *Ruin Nation: Destruction and the American Civil War*. Athens: University of Georgia Press, 2012.

Nielsen, Kim E. *A Disability History of the United States*. Boston: Beacon Street, 2012.

Padilla, Jalynn Olsen. "Army of 'Cripples': Civil War Amputees, Disability and Manhood in Victorian America." PhD diss., University of Delaware, 2007.

Pettegrew, John. *Brutes in Suits: Male Sensibility in America, 1890–1920*. Baltimore: Johns Hopkins University Press, 2007.

Powell, David A. *The Chickamauga Campaign: A Mad Irregular Battle; From the Crossing of the Tennessee River through the Second Day, August 22–September 19, 1863*. El Dorado Hills, CA: Savas Beatie, 2014.

Prokopowicz, Gerald J. *All for The Regiment: The Army of the Ohio, 1861–62*. Chapel Hill: University of North Carolina Press, 2001.

Pullen, John J. *Joshua Chamberlain: A Hero's Life and Legacy*. Mechanicsburg, PA: Stackpole Books, 1999.

Rajoppi, Joanne Hamilton, ed. *New Brunswick and the Civil War: The Brunswick Boys in the Great Rebellion*. Charleston: History Press, 2013.

Ramold, Steven J. *Baring the Iron Hand: Discipline in the Union Army*. DeKalb: University of Northern Illinois, 2009.

Reagan, Leslie J. "'My Daughter Was Genetically Drafted with Me': US-Vietnam War Veterans, Disabilities and Gender." *Gender & History* 28 (November 2016): 833–53.

Rembis, Michael. "Athlete First: A Note on Passing, Disability, and Sport," in *Disability and Passing: Blurring the Lines of Identity*, edited by Jeffrey A. Brune and Daniel J. Wilson, 111–41. Philadelphia: Temple University Press, 2013.

Rembis, Michael, and Susan Burch, eds. *Disability Histories*. Urbana: University of Illinois Press, 2014.

Riley, John P. "'This Is the Last Time I Shall Ever Leave My Family': Fatherhood in Civil War America." PhD diss., Binghamton University, 2017.
Rosenberg, Charles. *The Care of Strangers: The Rise of America's Hospital System.* New York: Basic Books, 1987.
Rotundo, E. Anthony. *American Manhood: Transformations in Masculinity from the Revolution to the Modern Era.* New York: Basic Books, 1993.
Rutkow, Ira. *Bleeding Blue and Gray: Civil War Surgery and the Evolution of American Medicine.* New York: Random House, 2005.
———. *Seeking the Cure: The History of American Medicine.* New York: Simon and Schuster, 2010.
Sappol, Michael. *A Traffic in Dead Bodies: Anatomy and Embodied Social Identity in Nineteenth-Century America.* Princeton, NJ: Princeton University Press, 2002.
Savitt, Todd. *Medicine and Slavery: The Diseases and Health Care of Blacks in Antebellum Virginia.* Urbana-Champaign: University of Illinois Press, 1981.
Schantz, Mark. *Awaiting the Heavenly Country: The Civil War and America's Culture of Death.* Ithaca, NY: Cornell University Press, 2008.
Schroeder-Lein, Glenna R. *The Encyclopedia of Civil War Medicine.* London: Routledge, 2015.
Schultz, Jane. *Women at the Front: Hospital Workers in Civil War America.* Chapel Hill: University of North Carolina Press, 2004.
Sears, Stephen W., ed. *Mr. Dunn Browne's Experiences in the Army: The Civil War Letters of Samuel W. Fiske.* New York: Fordham University Press, 1998.
Sellers, Charles. *The Market Revolution: Jacksonian America, 1815–1846.* Oxford: Oxford University Press, 1991.
Shaffer, Donald R. *After the Glory: The Struggles of Black Civil War Veterans.* Lawrence: University of Kansas Press, 2004.
Shakespeare, Tom. "Debating Disability." *Journal of Medical Ethics* 34 (2008): 11–14.
———. *Disability Rights and Wrongs.* London: Routledge, 2006.
———. *Disability Rights and Wrongs Revisited.* London: Taylor and Francis Group, 2013.
Shapiro, Joseph. *No Pity: People with Disabilities Forging a New Civil Rights Movement.* New York: Three Rivers, 1993.
Sheehan-Dean, Aaron. *Why Confederates Fought: Family and Nation in Civil War Virginia.* Chapel Hill: University of North Carolina Press, 2007.
Siebers, Tobin. *Disability Theory.* Ann Arbor: University of Michigan Press, 2008.
Silkenat, David. *Moments of Despair: Suicide, Divorce and Debt in Civil War Era North Carolina.* Chapel Hill: University of North Carolina Press, 2011.
Skloot, Rebecca. *The Immortal Life of Henrietta Lacks.* New York: Crown, 2011.
Skocpol, Theda. *Protecting Soldiers and Mothers: The Political Origins of Social Policy in the United States.* Cambridge, MA: Harvard University Press, 1995.
Slout, William L. *Burnt Cork and Tambourines: A Source Book of Negro Minstrelsy.* Rockville, MD: Wildside, 2007.

Smith, Charles James. *History of the Town of Mont Vernon, New Hampshire*. Boston: Blanchard, 1907.

Smith, Diane Monroe, ed. *Chamberlain at Petersburg: "The Charge at Fort Hell, June 18, 1864."* Gettysburg, PA: Thomas Publications, 2004.

———. *Fanny & Joshua: The Enigmatic Lives of Frances Caroline Adams and Joshua Lawrence Chamberlain*. Gettysburg, PA: Thomas Publications, 1999.

Smith, Jeffrey Allen, and B. Christopher Freuh. "Suicide, Alcoholism, and Psychiatric Illness among Union Forces during the U.S. Civil War." *Journal of Anxiety Disorders* 26 (2012): 769–75.

Smith, Michael Thomas. *The Enemy Within: Fears of Corruption in the Civil War North*. Richmond: University of Virginia Press, 2011.

Smith, Timothy B. *A Chickamauga Memorial: The Establishment of America's First Civil War National Military Park*. Knoxville: University of Tennessee Press, 2009.

Snyder, Katherine V. *Bachelors, Manhood, and the Novel, 1850–1925*. Oxford: Cambridge University Press, 1999.

Solomon, Zehava. *Combat Stress Reaction: The Enduring Toll of War*. New York: Spring Science + Business Media, 1993.

Sommerville, Diane Miller. *Aberration of Mind: Suicide and Suffering in the Civil War Era South*. Chapel Hill: University of North Carolina Press, 2018.

———. "'A Burden Too Heavy to Bear': War Trauma, Suicide, and Confederate Soldiers." *Civil War History* 59 (December 2013): 453–91.

———. "Will They Ever Be Able to Forget? Confederate Soldiers and Mental Illness in the Defeated South," in *Weirding the War: Stories from the Civil War's Ragged Edges*, edited by Stephen Berry, 321–39. Athens: University of Georgia Press, 2011.

Starr, Paul. *The Social Transformation of American Medicine*. New York: Basic Books, 1982.

Sternhell, Yael A. "Revisionism Reinvented? The Antiwar Turn in Civil War Scholarship." *Journal of the Civil War Era* 3 (2013): 239–56.

Summers, Mark Wahlgren. *The Press Gang: Newspapers and Politics, 1865–1878*. Chapel Hill: University of North Carolina Press, 1994.

———. *Rum, Romanism, & Rebellion: The Making of a President, 1884*. Chapel Hill: University of North Carolina Press, 2000.

Suplick, Stanley M., Jr. "The United States Invalid Corps / Veteran Reserve Corps." PhD diss., University of Minnesota, 1969.

Taylor, Amy Murrell. *The Divided Family in Civil War America*. Chapel Hill: University of North Carolina, 2005.

Tomes, Nancy. *The Art of Asylum-Keeping: Thomas Story Kirkbride and the Origins of American Psychiatry*. Philadelphia: University of Pennsylvania Press, 1994.

Trulock, Alice Rains. *In the Hands of Providence: Joshua Lawrence Chamberlain & the American Civil War*. Chapel Hill: University of North Carolina Press, 1992.

Ural, Susannah. *Don't Hurry Me Down to Hades: The Civil War in the Words of Those Who Lived It*. Oxford: Osprey, 2013.

Walsh, Chris. "'Cowardice, Weakness or Infirmity, Whichever It May Be Termed': A Shadow History of the Civil War." *Civil War History* 59 (December 2013): 492–526.

Washington, Harriet A. *Medical Apartheid: The Dark History of Medical Experimentation on Black Americans from Colonial Times to the Present*. New York: Doubleday, 2006.

Weitz, Mark A. *A Higher Duty: Desertion among Georgia Troops during the Civil War*. Lincoln: University of Nebraska Press, 2000.

———. *More Damning Than Slaughter: Desertion in the Confederate Army*. Lincoln: University of Nebraska Press, 2005.

Wendell, Susan. "Unhealthy Disabled: Treating Chronic Illnesses as Disabilities." *Hypatia* 16 (2001): 17–33.

Whitaker, Robert. *Mad in America: Bad Science, Bad Medicine, and the Enduring Mistreatment of the Mentally Ill*. New York: Perseus, 2002.

Whites, LeeAnn. *The Civil War as a Crisis in Gender: Augusta, Georgia, 1860–1890*. Athens: University of Georgia Press, 2000.

Whooley, Owen. *Knowledge in the Time of Cholera: The Struggle over American Medicine in the Nineteenth Century*. Chicago: University of Chicago Press, 2013.

Wilentz, Sean. *The Rise of American Democracy: Jefferson to Lincoln*. New York: W. W. Norton, 2005.

Wiley, Bell Irvin. *The Life of Billy Yank: The Common Soldier of the Union*. Baton Rouge: Louisiana State University Press, 1952.

Wise, Stephen R. *Gate of Hell: Campaign for Charleston Harbor, 1863*. Columbia: University of South Carolina Press, 1994.

Wu, Cynthia. *Chang and Eng Reconnected: The Original Siamese Twins in American Culture*. Philadelphia: Temple University Press, 2012.

INDEX

Abbott, Jenny, 79, 152n35
able-bodiedness, 6, 18, 34, 74, 83–84, 151n15; as critical to manhood, 17, 75, 87, 92, 121; presumptions of, 16, 22, 96, 103, 134; projection of, 13, 75, 78, 104. *See also* nondisabled people; passing (as able-bodied)
absenteeism, 35–37, 39, 98. *See also* desertion; leave
accommodation, 5, 7, 8, 10, 38, 79; as sign of weakness, 31, 34, 46
Act to Grant Pensions (1862), 20, 96
Adams, George, 78–79
addiction, 4, 27, 108, 111–12
Ames, Mary Clemmer, 59, 60, 67, 69, 147n39
amputation, 20–22, 104, 112, 129, 147n36, 151n14; as symbolic of patriotic sacrifice, 8, 53, 58–59, 85, 88; as typical Civil War wound, 13, 19, 34, 67, 84–85, 133; as visible disability, 2, 17, 47, 74–75
amputees, 82–84, 88, 134
anatomical specimens, 52, 56–58, 62, 64, 68, 147n27
Anderson, Benjamin, 65–67, 69, 149n61
Army Medical Department, 18, 57, 64, 68–69, 133; medical directors in, 11, 23, 66; use of soldiers' bodies by, 8, 52–54, 56, 61–62. *See also* Brinton, John
Army Medical Museum, 8, 51–52, 56–62, 67–69, 154n75
Arrears Act (1879), 96
Articles of War, 19, 33, 34, 38, 142n1
autopsy, 52, 55, 65–67, 147n22, 149n64

Barnum, Henry A., 69, 70, 88–92
Barnum, P. T., 63, 64

Bartholow, Roberts, 14–15, 18, 43–44, 48, 98
Battle of Chickamauga, 81, 111
Battle of Fredericksburg, 11, 58, 71, 107–8, 118, 126, 138n1
Battle of Gettysburg, 41, 71, 119; 126; injury of Dan Sickles at, 40, 59; and Joshua Chamberlain, 79, 92
beggary. *See* pauperism
Bellard, Alfred, 16, 22
Belt, Rabia, 3
Billings, John Shaw, 57, 59, 67
Black, John C., 107, 155n2
blacks, 12–14, 28–30, 61, 105, 141n76; bodies of, 56, 65–66, 69, 142n79, 149n68
Blanck, Peter, 104, 105
blindness, 19, 44, 86, 97, 104
bodies, 2–3, 29, 30, 133; authority over, as contested, 13, 18–19, 52–54, 119, 121; of blacks, 56, 65–66, 69, 142n79, 149n68; display of, 63–66, 68–69; and medicine, role in advancing, 8, 52, 55–57, 61–63, 84; as property of the state, 12, 49, 51; and white manhood, 34–39, 45, 51–52, 103–4, 134. *See also* autopsy; corpses; war wounds
Bourne, William Oland, 83
Bowdoin College, 73, 82, 86
Boynton, Henry Van Ness, 68–69, 81, 149n73
brain injury, 1, 58–59, 131
Brennan, Murty, 106
Brenton, William (pseud.), 126, 162n42
Brinton, John, 51, 52, 56; collection of specimens by, 57–58, 62, 69, 147n27. *See also* Army Medical Museum
Brown, Edgar (pseud.), 122
Brunswick (Maine), 80, 81, 82, 86
Busby, James V., 97

cadavers. *See* corpses
camps: for convalescents, 11, 16, 17, 138n22; diseases in, 7, 20, 88, 110, 133; for prisoners of war, 29, 102, 122
casualties. *See* war wounds
Chamberlain, Fanny, 86; allegations of domestic violence by, 80–81; ignorance of husband's condition, 83; marriage with Joshua, altered by injury, 79–80, 82, 116, 152n38
Chamberlain, Joshua Lawrence, 4, 8, 89, 134, 150n11; medical treatment of, 76–79, 83–84; and passing as nondisabled, 5, 73–75, 78–79, 85–86, 92–94; and struggles surrounding pension, 86–88, 104, 105, 154n78; suffering of, during service, 71–73, 151n19, 152n37, 153n48; wound's impact on marriage of, 79–82, 116, 151n25, 152n38
Chickamauga. *See* Battle of Chickamauga
Cimbala, Paul, 14, 17, 150n13
Circular No. 2, 54, 56, 62
citizenship, 4, 12, 29
citizen-soldiers, 8, 13, 40, 62, 73, 96; ideals used in judgment of, 3–4, 47–49, 98–99, 103, 107. *See also* soldiers
Civil War, 2–4, 137n11; impact on soldiers' families, 116, 132; and medical science, 9–10, 39–40, 48, 51–53, 56–57; race relations during, 28–29; and wounded soldiers, 12, 75, 88, 120, 133–35
Clarke, Frances, 13, 40, 45, 48, 74
class, 48, 55–56, 143n8, 156n38; as linked with manhood, 3, 13, 35, 75, 103–4
Cleveland, Grover, 155n2, 158n58, 158n71; doubting of veterans by, 110–11, 112–14; and mistrust of pension system, 106–7, 109–10; and pension vetoes, 9, 95, 99, 108
Confederacy, 36, 58, 69, 71, 100–102
Confederate soldiers: as model veterans, 100–101, 151n17; purported barbarity of, 25, 61, 69, 102, 117
Conover, William, 66–67
conscripts, 14, 22, 98
convalescence, 14–18, 45, 138n22
Cornell, Alonzo, 92
corpses, 49, 57, 69; of soldiers, medical use for, 53, 54–55, 65–66
Costa, Dora, 7, 153n48, 156n32

courts-martial, 6, 134, 142n1, 146n8; of army surgeon, for autopsy, 62–67; and defining disability, 37–39; and malingering, 41, 44; of sick soldiers, 7–8, 33–34, 46–47, 49
cowardice, 12, 48; impairment perceived as, 16, 27, 35–36, 37, 43–44, 143n11; and pension debates, 101, 102, 109, 112; *See also* absenteeism; malingering
craniometry, 61, 148n42

Danielson, Charles (pseud.), 120–21, 160n21
Davis, Cyrus, 104
Davis, N. Ann, 74
Davis, Zechariah, 105
DeForest, John W., 17, 24, 25, 139n36, 141n58
Democrats, 16, 96, 107, 113
Dempsey, Marshall, 65, 66
dependency, 121; of disabled soldiers, solutions for addressing, 7, 20–21, 87–88, 124–25; and masculinity, 4, 12–13, 101, 134; racialization of, 12–13, 29–30; stigma of, 3–4, 5, 123. *See also* labor; self-sufficiency
Dependent Pension Bill, 99–100
deserters, as unworthy veterans, 101–2
desertion, 16, 35–36, 98, 103, 113; and military's changing policies concerning, 36, 143n8; pension cases, 101–3, 120–21; as precipitated by impairment, 37–38, 44, 134, 143n7
detachment (clinical), 52, 57–58
Devine, Shauna, 52
disability, 2–3, 5–7, 12, 37, 134; as defined by capacity for labor, 30, 95–97; degrees of disability, 7, 29, 59, 94, 109; and emasculating dependency, 4, 103, 104–7, 118, 120–21, 125; government's role in determining, 17–18, 22, 86–87, 104–6; interpersonal consequences of, 81–82, 115–17, 124–32; legitimacy of, debates over, 9, 34–37, 44–47, 109; overcoming of, 5, 75, 84–85, 87, 123; racialization of, 12, 18–19, 29, 105. *See also* able-bodiedness; mental disability; nondisabled people; nonvisible disability
disability discharge, 2, 48, 105, 119, 122, 144n26; from chronic illness, 7, 14–15, 34–36, 95; difficulty obtaining, 17, 33, 42
disabled people, 3–4, 49, 92–93, 134;

assumptions about, 6, 9, 151n19, 152n38, 159n5; difficulties faced by, 5, 74, 113, 151n15
discipline, 16, 19, 35, 47, 66, 139n22
disease. *See* illness
dishonorable discharge, 67, 98, 101, 134, 156n32. *See also* unworthy veterans
Dodge, John, 97
Donnelly, Edward, 63–64, 65, 67
drunkenness, 22, 27, 47, 126, 147n27
Duffy, James, 59
Dunn, Walter, 23–24

Ellis, Benjamin, 120, 127
Ellis, Mary, 127
emasculation, 9, 12, 70, 74–77, 81
"The Empty Sleeve" (song), 85
enlistment, 18, 21, 34, 51, 54, 138n7; controversies surrounding, 14, 26, 98–99, 101
Enrollment Act, 14

Farnum, George, 11, 15, 16, 23
Faust, Drew Gilpin, 55
federal pension system. *See* Pension Bureau
First Battalion (of Invalid Corps), 22, 24
fitness for field service, 7, 41, 48, 79, 139n37; determination of, 33–34, 39–41; doubts surrounding, 14–18, 36. *See also* disability discharge
Folsom, Daniel (pseud.), 117–18, 132
Foote, Lorien, 3
Fredericksburg. *See* Battle of Fredericksburg
Fry, James B., 20, 26
furlough. *See* leave

Garfield, James, 89–92
General Order 36, 15
General Order 61, 36
General Order 65, 36, 42
General Order 105, 17, 139n37
General Order 111, 26
General Order 143, 14
General Order 212, 17–18, 139n37
genital trauma, 76–77, 81–82, 134
Gettysburg. *See* Battle of Gettysburg
Godding, W. W., 128, 130
Gordon (enslaved person), 29–30
Grand Army of the Republic, 96, 99, 107

Gray, John P., 119, 120, 122
Green, Alfred, 60
Greenberg, Amy, 3
Griggs, Abraham P., 95–96, 107–9, 134

Hammond, William A., 18, 54–55, 62
Harrison, Simon, 58
Hatton, William H. D., 62–64
Hayes, Franklin B., 128–29
Holmes, Oliver Wendell, Sr., 84, 86
Hood, John Bell, 82
Humphreys, Margaret, 15

idleness, 15, 20, 24, 122
illness: bodily suffering caused by, 38–40, 46–48, 83, 86–87; categorization of, as a disability, 7, 74–79, 109–10, 142n5; military violations precipitated by, 37–42; skepticism of, 35–36, 43–46, 98, 102; ubiquity of, 18–20, 151n14. *See also* infection; "walking sick"
"imbecility," 19, 95, 108
independence. *See* self-sufficiency
infection, 23, 59, 92, 153n48; as chronic condition, 7, 73, 77, 82, 105, 112 *See also* illness; war wounds
Ingram, Thomas, 87
injury. *See* war wounds
insanity. *See* mental disability
institutionalization, 9, 159n6, 160n8; and families, consequences for, 116, 124–30; soldiers' hardships during, 118–20, 121–22, 122–24. *See also* mental disability
Invalid Corps, 7–8, 11–12, 106, 124, 140n44; as alternative to dependency, 7, 12, 20, 104; as efficient use of military resources, 14–21, 22–23, 30, 51, 139n37; racial politics of, 28–31; soldiers' attitudes toward, 23–25, 26–28, 34, 36. *See also* Veteran Reserve Corps
"The Invalid Corps" (song), 26–28
Invalid Corps officers, 19, 20, 25, 27, 139n41

Johnson, Geoffrey (pseud.), 126, 162n38
Jones, Jonathan, 4
Jordan, Brian Matthew, 53, 96

Kielhoffer, Francis, 125, 126
Kielhoffer, Maria, 125, 126

Kyle, Jacob (pseud.), 126, 162n40
Kyle, Joanna Nicholls, 61

labor: as factor in defining disability, 3–4, 20–22, 104–5, 120–22, 125, 139n38; military's deficiency in, 7, 12, 14–15; military's preservation of, 15–19, 21–22, 29, 108; as remedy for illness, 15, 33, 108, 118, 122. *See also* productivity
leave, 16, 34, 72, 76, 82; in form of furlough, 14, 36–38, 46, 143n11; in form of sick leave, 36, 49. *See also* absenteeism; disability discharge
light duty, 15, 33, 36–37, 41, 46
Lincoln, Abraham, 14, 36, 155n1
Linderman, Gerald, 4
Lockwood, George, 89
Logue, Larry, 105

madness. *See* mental disability
Maine, 73, 79, 80–81, 83, 87
malingerers, 25–27, 41, 47–49, 95, 98
malingering, 11, 16, 41–44, 113; as a deficiency in manhood, 34–35, 45, 49, 102–3, 108–9; nonvisible disabilities and, 19, 42, 46, 74. *See also* "pluck"
Manderson, Charles F., 105–6
marriage, 80–82
Marten, James, 4, 97
Martin, Robert (pseud.), 121–22, 123, 124, 127, 161n24
masculinity: and dependency, 3–4, 12–13, 100–101, 123; impairment as deficiency in, 9, 33, 35, 40–41, 45–48; and light duty, 16–17, 28–30; military service as proof of, 12; and pension cases, 97, 102–6, 108–11, 112–13; rehabilitation of, 116, 121, 123
masturbation, 43, 122, 129, 161n26
McCall, George, 62–63
McGrogan, James, 41, 42, 44
McKinley, William, 92
McMorris, R. M., 108–9
McReynolds, Lizzie Wilson, 115–16, 130–32
Medal of Honor, 92, 107, 149n73
"The Medical and Surgical History of the War of the Rebellion" (MSHWR), 19, 39–42, 89, 140n44, 154n75
medical officers: duties of, during combat, 14–17, 18, 31, 40–42, 54; as gatekeepers to field service, 18, 36–39, 42–44, 95, 105, 139n37; procurement of anatomy specimens by, 52, 54–59, 62–65, 66–69; treatment of war wounds by, 11, 23, 72–73; as witnesses against soldiers, 33, 41, 43–44, 46–47, 87–88
medicine: sacrifices for, by war wounded, 51–53, 57–58, 61; war's contribution to advancement in, 1–3, 8, 53–56, 62–65, 83–86; and wartime controversy, 55–56, 65–67. *See also* Army Medical Department; Army Medical Museum; medical officers
memory, 8, 52–53, 64, 76, 127
mental disability, 9, 12, 59, 160n8, 161n31; and families of soldiers, 124–30, 132; physical activity as remedy for, 103–4, 122; skepticism toward, 110–13, 119; war's liability for, 115–17, 120, 123–24, 131, 132. *See also* war trauma
Mezurek, Kelly, 29
Millender, Michael, 104
Mitchell, Michael (pseud.), 126, 162n39
Mitchell, Reid, 4
Moncrief, John T., 128
Moore, Clinton (pseud.), 126–27, 162n43
Moss, Dr. William, 58, 145n1

Native Americans, 14, 56, 60–62
Neilsen, Kim, 5
New Hallowell Hospital, 11, 16, 23
New York, 22, 55, 123, 101, 117
New York Herald, 99, 100
New York State Lunatic Asylum (Utica, NY), 159n6, 160n8; soldiers' occupancy in, 117–19, 121, 123, 126–27, 132
New York Times, 82, 86
nondisabled people, 5, 25, 74–75, 87. *See also* able-bodiedness; passing
nonvisible disability, 2, 8–9, 83–84, 92–93, 104–5. *See also* passing
Norris, Jeremiah (pseud.), 122, 161n26
nostalgia, 99, 151n22; "morbid," medical diagnosis of, 43–46, 145n51, 145n52

O'Niel, John, 46–47, 49
Otis, George, 89
Owen, Annie, 109–10

Owen, Mortimer B., 109–10

Padilla, Jalynn Olsen, 103
pain, 3, 18, 23, 68, 152n38; expectations for bearing of, 9, 40–41, 48, 78, 87, 92, 108; as an impairment, 34, 39, 42, 73, 77–78, 82, 86, 93; nonvisiblity of, 42–43, 47, 74; opiate use to manage, 111–12; skepticism of, 6, 35, 43, 47–48, 113
Palmer, B. Frank, 84
passing (as able-bodied), 5, 13, 75, 78, 92. *See also* "pluck"; self-mastery
The Passing of the Armies (Chamberlain), 75
patriotism, 13, 42, 93, 98, 151n22; bodily sacrifices in the name of, 3, 8–9, 30, 62–63, 76, 85; manliness as measure of, 45, 69, 92, 100–102, 110, 134. *See also* citizen-soldiers
pauperism, 88; as antithetical to manhood, 3–4, 98, 100–101, 105–6, 121; Invalid Corps's role in preventing, 7, 21
Pelton, Ephraim, 33–34, 35, 39, 46, 48
pension appeals, 87–88, 95; and Cleveland vetoes, 106, 107–9, 110–13
Pension Bureau, 4, 6–9, 158n68; debates surrounding, 5, 20, 96–98; definitions of disability asserted by, 3, 105–6, 109, 111–13, 119; scrutiny by, to prevent fraud, 49, 86–89, 93, 95, 103–4
pension fraud, 96–98, 102–3, 107–9, 112–13
pensions, 3, 20–21, 104–5, 155n1, 157n51; politics of, 96–99, 102–3, 107–13; stigma surrounding, 12, 21, 100–102, 105–6, 110; veterans' pursuit of, 9, 49, 95–97, 101, 107–10
"pluck," 3, 40–41, 92, 100, 138n14; lack of, and malingering accusations, 41, 45–48. *See also* malingerers; malingering
Porter, Fitz John, 86, 87
Portland Oregonian, 99, 100
Portland Transcript, 83, 85
Potts, George, 64–67, 149n68
Potts, Jane, 110, 111
Potts, Noah, 110–11
poverty. *See* pauperism
Preston, Sally Buchanan, 82
productivity, 30; as measure of manhood, 4, 20, 124; used to define disability, 18, 104, 121. *See also* labor; self-sufficiency

prosthetics, 2, 84–85, 101, 131
psychological trauma. *See* war trauma
PTSD (post-traumatic stress disorder), 116, 159n3

race, 2, 28–30; and martial manhood, 12–14, 103; and treatment of soldiers' bodies, 52, 56, 61–62, 65–66, 148n46. *See also* blacks; whiteness
Ramold, Steven, 38, 143n7, 143n8
regiments: absenteeism within, 17, 38–39, 44; loyalty to, 11, 23–24, 30, 108; medical issues in, 13, 14, 16, 64–66
Rembis, Michael, 75
Republicans, 96, 99, 100, 106–7, 110
Reynolds, John F., 63, 64
rheumatism, 19, 33, 42–43, 95–96, 105–8
Roosevelt, Theodore, 103

sacrifice, 10, 73, 75–76, 131, 151n22; as patriotic duty, 2–3, 9, 13, 85, 93; of soldiers' bodies for science, 61–62, 69; visible disability as proof of, 47, 53, 83, 88. *See also* patriotism
Sartorius, Wrede, 1, 2, 8, 9
Scott, Harvey W., 99, 100
Seaborn, Isaiah (pseud.), 126, 162n38
Second Battalion (of Invalid Corps), 22, 24, 47
self-care, 35–39, 49, 105, 134
self-mastery, 3–4; as critical to able-bodied manhood, 13, 45, 75, 103. *See also* passing; "pluck"
self-sufficiency, 3–4, 104; institutionalized soldiers' desire for, 120, 121, 125; and war wounds, 12–13, 87. *See also* dependency; labor; productivity
Sewell, William Joyce, 110
shame, 23, 45, 102, 106, 109. *See also* stigma
Shaw, Robert Gould, 61, 148n46, 149n68
Shively, Kathryn, 35, 40
Sickles, Dan, 40, 59, 147n36
sickness. *See* illness
Siebers, Tobin, 87, 151n15
Simms, Albion, 1, 8–9
Sims, J. Marion, 66, 149n63
Skocpol, Theda, 74, 97, 156n36
Smith, Clinton, 111–12
Smith, Eliza, 111–12

soldiers (Union), 38, 62, 100, 132, 141n70, 142n3; during combat, 35–36, 42, 46–48. *See also* citizen-soldiers; Confederate soldiers; veterans
Sommerville, Diane Miller, 116
St. Elizabeths Hospital (Washington, DC), 115, 117, 120, 125–30, 159n6
Stanton, Edwin, 15, 17, 20, 29, 147n27
stigma, 7, 21, 25, 101; and disabled people, 3, 5, 23; and mental illness, 9, 118, 119, 122; and opiate use, 110–12. *See also* shame
Stockwell, John, 97
"straggling." *See* absenteeism
suicide, 110, 118, 122, 123, 126, 140n46. *See also* mental disability
"supercrip," 5, 137n10, 151n19
surgeons. *See* medical officers
syphilis, 19, 46

Tanner, James, 4, 105, 157n51
temperance, 3, 112. *See also* addiction; self-mastery
Thompson, William, 117
Toombs, Gregory (pseud.), 118–20, 121, 123, 124

Union army, 3–4; contested issues within, 29–31, 97–99; efficiency and strength of, 7–8, 14, 22–23; ideas of disability shaped by, 12, 20–21, 101; non-fatal casualties within, 34–37, 39–40, 43–44, 138n1, 144n26. *See also* citizen-soldiers; regiments; soldiers (Union); veterans (Union)
United States Colored Troops (USCT), 14, 28–29, 64, 66, 69, 105
unworthy veterans, 88, 95–98, 112–13; deserters as, 101–2; malingerers as, 102–3; mercenaries as, 98–101. *See also* malingerers; pension appeals; pension fraud

"The Veteran" (poem), 85

Veteran Reserve Corps (VRC), 7, 11, 24, 26, 106, 140n43. *See also* Invalid Corps
veterans (Union), 2, 3–5, 13; ambivalence toward, 88, 97–98, 103–5, 109–13; support solicited by, 9–10, 49, 88, 92, 98–99, 106–7; unrealistic expectations of, 53, 74–75, 81–83, 85, 99–101; war's emotional toll on, 69–70, 116–17, 123–24. *See also* citizen-soldiers; Confederate soldiers; unworthy veterans

"walking sick," 7, 8, 31, 33–37, 49, 51
War Department, 3, 7, 12, 14–18, 21, 36
Warren, Joseph H., 82, 83, 84, 85, 86
war trauma, 9, 87, 109, 133–34; social consequences of, 113, 115–17, 124–27, 128–32, 159n3. *See also* mental disability
war wounds, 19–20, 59–60, 79, 82–83, 88–92; long-term complications from, 69–70, 72–73, 106, 109–12, 150n11; social consequences of, 18, 34–35, 79–81, 116; suspected legitimacy of, 2–3, 8–9, 122–23, 132; symbolism of, 13, 30, 134, 151n14. *See also* disability; illness
Washington Star, 67, 68
whiteness, 29–30, 61, 66; as central to manhood, 12–13, 51, 75, 103–4. *See also* race
Whites, LeeAnn, 12
Wilder, Frank, 26–28
Wiley, Bell, 40
Willard Asylum for the Chronic Insane (Ovid, NY), 117, 123, 126, 159n6, 160n8, 162n38
willpower. *See* self-mastery
Wilson, David, 131
Wilson, John, 115, 130
work. *See* labor

Young, Michael, 47, 49

Zane, Harriet, 125
Zane, Joseph, 125

UnCivil Wars

Weirding the War: Stories from the Civil War's Ragged Edges
    EDITED BY STEPHEN BERRY

Ruin Nation: Destruction and the American Civil War
    BY MEGAN KATE NELSON

America's Corporal: James Tanner in War and Peace
    BY JAMES MARTEN

The Blue, the Gray, and the Green:
Toward an Environmental History of the Civil War
    EDITED BY BRIAN ALLEN DRAKE

Empty Sleeves: Amputation in the Civil War South
    BY BRIAN CRAIG MILLER

Lens of War: Exploring Iconic Photographs of the Civil War
    EDITED BY J. MATTHEW GALLMAN AND GARY W. GALLAGHER

The Slave-Trader's Letter-Book: Charles Lamar, the Wanderer,
and Other Tales of the African Slave Trade
    BY JIM JORDAN

Driven from Home: North Carolina's Civil War Refugee Crisis
    BY DAVID SILKENAT

The Ghosts of Guerrilla Memory: How Civil War Bushwhackers Became
Gunslingers in the American West
    BY MATTHEW CHRISTOPHER HULBERT

Beyond Freedom: Disrupting the History of Emancipation
    EDITED BY DAVID W. BLIGHT AND JIM DOWNS

The Lost President: A. D. Smith and the Hidden History of Radical
Democracy in Civil War America
    BY RUTH DUNLEY

Bodies in Blue: Disability in the Civil War North
    BY SARAH HANDLEY-COUSINS

Household War: How Americans Lived and Fought the Civil War
    EDITED BY LISA TENDRICH FRANK AND LEEANN WHITES

Lightning Source UK Ltd.
Milton Keynes UK
UKHW042143200619
344772UK00001B/61/P